PARTNER
YOGA

PARTNER YOGA

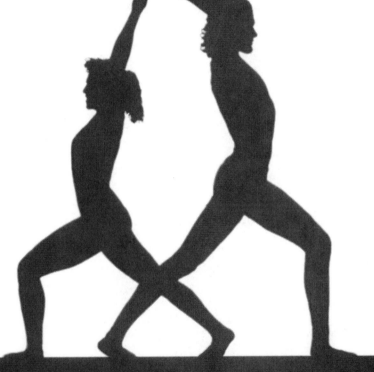

Making Contact for Physical, Emotional, and Spiritual Growth

Cain Carroll and Lori Kimata, N.D.

An Imprint of Rodale Books

Notice

If you have a serious injury or illness, consult a health professional before practicing Partner Yoga. Not all the exercises and poses are suitable for everyone, and this or any exercise program could result in injury. To reduce the risk of injury, do not force or strain. Pregnant women are advised not to practice twisting poses or any exercise that places strain on the abdomen. Women who are menstruating are advised not to practice inverted poses or poses that place heavy pressure on the abdomen. When in doubt, always consult a competent health professional.

Cover Designer: Christopher Rhoads
Interior Designers: Christopher Rhoads and Susan P. Eugster
Cover Photographer: Ken Gray

Library of Congress Cataloging-in-Publication Data

Carroll, Cain.
    Partner yoga : making contact for physical, emotional, and spiritual growth / Cain Carroll and Lori Kimata.
        p.   cm.
    Includes bibliographical references (p.   ) and index.
    ISBN: 978-1-60529-699-9
    1. Yoga, Hatha.   I. Kimata, Lori.   II. Title.
  RA781.7 .C388   2000
  613.7'046—dc21   00–059227

Distributed to the book trade by St. Martin's Press

6 8 10 9 7 5   paperback

Visit us on the Web at www.rodalebooks.com, or call us toll-free at (800) 848-4735.

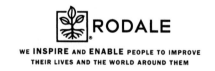

WE **INSPIRE** AND **ENABLE** PEOPLE TO IMPROVE
THEIR LIVES AND THE WORLD AROUND THEM

TO THE TRUTH FINDERS

Contents

Part Three: Expanding Beyond

Foreword

Health has become a big business and a frequent topic in the media. It is not uncommon to hear about people having nutritional deficiencies of vitamins, minerals, and the important types of dietary fatty acids. There are two deficiencies we rarely hear discussed, however. This book is about these two deficiencies: A lack of quality movement and a lack of quality touch, and a means to remedy the lack of these in your life. The integration of these two very basic needs in a system called Partner Yoga, presented in this book, gives you a new tool to meet the basic requirements for good health.

Yoga conjures up a variety of images in people's minds. Yet at its core, yoga is really quite simple to understand. The physical practice of yoga is a complete system of physical exercise and healthy movement that integrates balance, flexibility, grace, and strength. Yoga is about exploring the boundaries of your current limitations and eventually moving through these limitations. At its essence, yoga is the state of perfect harmony of body, mind, and spirit.

We are all familiar with stress and recognize that consistent, elevated levels of it are not in keeping with our best health interests. After 17 years in private medical practice, I can assure you that a chronically high level of stress is a recipe for a health disaster. So any tool you can bring to bear that either reduces stress or allows you to manage it more effectively is always a great health investment. The regular practice of yoga provides just such an opportunity.

Studies consistently show that yoga has significant anti-stress benefits. As a rule, people who choose to practice yoga have much more balanced moods and a higher degree of satisfaction with their lives. They become less excitable, less aggressive, and less anxious. They will tell you that they have a better sense of well-being, more consistent feelings of relaxation, improved concentration, greater self-confidence, improved efficiency, better interpersonal relationships, increased attentiveness, lowered irritability levels, and a more optimistic outlook on the events shaping their lives.

Changes in your ability to handle stress can be measured in the levels of stress hormones that you create. Over time with the consistent practice of yoga, the levels of these stress hormones will begin to normalize. Yoga's anti-stress effects can be monitored by looking at your nervous system—it becomes more balanced.

Another key aspect of health centers around improving certain functional markers. These provide a portrait of your actual biological age, which, from a health perspective, is much more important than your chronological age. Some of the most important markers for health include muscle mass, strength, aerobic capacity, body fat, bone density, posture, cholesterol levels, blood pressure, and the tendency for platelets to aggregate or be "sticky." Yoga actually promotes consistent improvement in all of these functional markers.

We all know intuitively that touch transmits a true sense of caring and generates a form of nourishment that cannot be captured in any other manner. If you doubt the power of touch, imagine the sensation of an embrace with a dear friend or spouse or the sensation after someone gives you a massage.

When animals are deprived of touch or contact, they inevitably get sick or develop psychological disturbances. At one unfortunate point in the history of health care, the standard was to deprive newborns of human contact immediately following birth. Fortunately, this trend was reversed, but only after astute observers noticed the effects that touch deprivation had on health. It is no secret that many self-help and addiction-recovery groups emphasize hugging as a regular ritual of their meetings. This is intentional—many people are deficient in the key area of human touch.

Nothing can replace the need for consistent, quality human touch. We derive nourishment from touch just as we derive nourishment from the food we choose to eat.

As a second-generation naturopathic doctor, I was exposed to and involved with many aspects of nonconventional medicine from an early age. The system of Partner Yoga that Cain Carroll and Lori Kimata, N.D., have created is a valuable contribution to the library of integrative medicine.

When I ask my patients to make changes in their eating habits and lifestyle, I always emphasize the need to give something a try and measure its value by experiencing the result. I lay the same challenge before you, dear reader: Read this book, try the strategies, and experience the difference in your life.

—PETER D'ADAMO, N.D.
AUTHOR OF *EAT RIGHT FOR YOUR TYPE*

Acknowledgments

We extend our heartfelt appreciation to everyone who has helped bring this project to fruition. Special thanks to our photographer, Ken Gray, who has the uncanny ability to capture the visual essence of Partner Yoga and the energy to climb mountains to get the shot. To our literary agent, Debra Goldstein, for believing in us from the beginning and propelling us forward with unfailing enthusiasm. This project would not have been possible without our editor, Nancy Hancock, our publisher, Neil Wertheimer, and all the wonderful folks at Rodale who breathed life into these pages. Sincere thanks to Dr. Greg Kelly and Dr. Peter D'Adamo for their support in writing our foreword. To all those who gave their time and energy during the photo shoots: Neal Oppen for driving, lifting, and doing everything the rest of us were too tired to do; Annie Dubois for keeping us aligned; Andrea Torres for her artistic direction and moral support; and Cherie and Tesa DeHaven, Arn Phillips, Tirrell McGrueder, Maile Labasan and Jesse Parungao, Fely Ebner, Berton Wong, and Jason and Brian Govreau for modeling our poses. Thank you also to John Signor and Andrea Torres for opening their home to us during the Maui photo shoot. Kudos to Cotton Cargo and Busy Bodies (in Honolulu) for discounting the outfits we wore in the photos. Warm thanks to Dad and Jean for letting us soak our sore muscles in their hot tub.

From Cain: I am deeply grateful to my family for their continual support, acceptance, and unconditional love; to Das for creating a space where true yoga is lived, rain or shine, 7 days a week; to Rich McCord and the staff at the

Expanding Light for gently persisting that I take my practice deeper, and deeper still; to Cheryl Flaharty for pushing me to new frontiers in body, mind, and spirit; to The Iona Pears for accepting me into the ohana and inspiring me with their radiance and authenticity; to my friend and mentor, Gavan Daws, for sharing green tea ice cream and invaluable counsel on how to become an author; to Norbert Larson for sharing space and putting up with an office in the living room; to John Signor for believing in me and listening to first drafts with an encouraging smile and eager ears; to Nine-Toes for reminding me to laugh hard and live true; to Monte Gores for keeping the friendship alive and growing; and to my yoga students for taking the journey with me. Finally, thank you to the countless other souls who have influenced and inspired this project in so many ways. Sat Nam.

From Lori: Deep gratitude to Mom and Dad for having the courage to bring me into this world, and to my family for always standing by my side; to Cain and Ken, my buddies and true partners who care and trust so much; to Donny, who showed me my first partner posture and opened my heart to such love and joy, and to Gurudez and Das for keeping that bright light of yoga burning before me; to *all* of you amazing souls who have taught me about life, love, and intimacy—you know who you are—the lessons have been challenging and the teachers many. Gratitude also to Jack, for helping me up when I fall and for always being there for me; to all my students who have trusted me and all the moms who have taught me so much about patience and surrender; to Lynn, Mala, Marianne, Annie, and Das for getting my being ready for the photos in this book; to Louise, Lawrence, Pete, Heather, Samar, Nine-Toes, and all the Colorado folks who walked those early pre-labor Partner Yoga book miles with me; to Elizabeth, Harriet, Dan, Sarah, Medra, Ann, Cathie, Teri, Natasha, Erik, and Craig, who keep teaching me to love passionately, cry fully, and play forever; and to Dhira, Seguin, Reggae, Orlando, Michel, Lansana, Kapono, and all the great musicians and dancers who keep inspiring me to listen carefully and dance wildly . . . and especially to that little voice inside me whose patience and persistence has kept me so fully alive . . . I am so deeply grateful to you all, and to everyone who has touched my life. Sat Nam.

Introduction: How It All Began

"The skin is no more separated from the brain than the surface of a lake is separate from its depths; the two are different locations in a continuous medium . . . The brain is a single functional unit, from cortex to fingertips to toes. To touch the surface is to stir the depths."

—Deane Juhan, Trager specialist

The sun set over the desert as heat from the ground met the sky in a brilliant display of color. Silhouettes of cactus and creosote meshed together on the horizon as twilight approached. Outdoor life commenced with the sunset, as the evening brought relief from the scorching heat.

It was a full moon, and a variety of people gathered at the local park just a step away from Phoenix's sprawling cement jungle. About 30 people had crawled out of their city lives to form a drumming circle and commune with nature. Half of the people were playing instruments, a few kids were running around, and a dozen men and women were shaking wildly to the entrancing music.

On this warm Arizona night many full moons ago, our paths first touched. We had each managed to clear some space in our schedules to spend this auspicious evening in the park. Most of the drummers seemed to know each other at least by first name. Since both of us had arrived after the drumming had started, we missed the initial introduction. Fortunately, we were used to drum circles, so we jumped right in and drummed passionately for the next few hours. Finally, the music climaxed and fell into a soothing silence as people laid down their instruments and relaxed into the cooling grass.

Cain: *When I met Lori, I was a student at Arizona State working toward my degree in intercultural communication. To balance the stress of my academic pursuits, I spent part of my free time practicing hand drum rhythms with local drummers. Every month, I would join the full moon drum circle. Unlike the sometimes confining structure of the university, a drum circle thrives on improvisation and total freedom of expression. Under the full moon there are no rules, there is no curriculum, and everyone is equal. The music is raw and primitive, and it brings people closer to themselves and each other. Inhibitions dissolve and people are real. I couldn't have staged a more perfect place to meet the person with whom I would co-create a project about truth, partnership, and interdependence.*

Lori: *I had almost decided to leave drumming behind me in Hawaii. It was hard to leave the drum troupe I had been playing with for a few years, and I didn't know if I was ready for a new scene. My life was starting to fill up again, even though I was doing my best to keep it simple. Besides my naturopathic medical practice and midwifery practice, I was teaching a number of classes in the community and at the naturopathic college. I had taken a break from my years of teaching yoga in Hawaii and was practicing on my own, except for an occasional class and a few private clients. My yoga practice was deepening*

and I felt ready for something new. I sensed something big shifting into gear in my life. People were always asking me why I moved from the beauty of Hawaii to the desolation of the desert. There was a solitude I found there. The desert allowed me the space and time to sift through the multitude of amazing gifts life had afforded me. It was a time for me to go inward. Yet that night, something drew me outward, just far enough to make it to the park, despite my stack of paperwork and all the phone calls I needed to return. Fortunately, I listened to my intuitive voice.

Everyone was unwinding in their own way. We noticed each other moving through different yoga postures in the changing shadows. Without words, we began extending toward each other, reaching out and stretching into mutually supportive new yoga postures together. We could sense where the other person needed support or encouragement. We both experienced a fuller stretch and a deeper sense of relaxation. We were having fun and creating something more than either of us could create alone. It felt natural to blend our yoga practices.

Then our minds kicked in and our inhibitions surfaced. "What am I doing? I don't even know this person! Is this really appropriate? I wonder who's watching?" We caught each other's apprehensive looks and cracked up. Laughter broke the tension and we relaxed and let go. Both of us were giving into and gaining from this dynamic and playful experience. As our minds relaxed more, our hearts opened and our bodies flowed with greater ease. We brought our newly joined

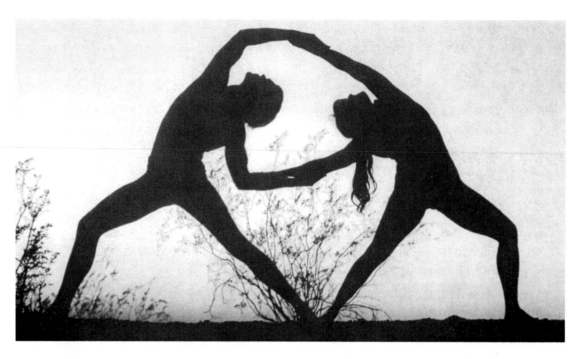

practice to a close and rested in the stillness of the starlit desert night. Truly connecting with another human being had reawakened our spirits in a completely new way.

Lori: *My good friends know that when I get excited about something, I put my energy into it 110 percent. That's what happened with my new yoga practice with Cain. It was the perfect next step for me. It integrated naturopathic medicine with my love for creative dance, contact improvisation, art, spontaneity, partnership, fitness, fun, relaxation, intimacy, and of course, yoga. I have always been a "touchy" person—and practicing yoga "in touch" with another person was just what I needed.*

Excited about our new art form, which we dubbed Partner Yoga, we furthered our commitment by creating space for it in our lives. As our friendship grew, we began to practice three or four times a week, integrating partner work into our already existing yoga and exercise programs. Soon we were practicing partner postures wherever we happened to be—in the rock climbing gym, at the park after work, before or after teaching other yoga classes. We introduced Partner Yoga to our friends, family, and even strangers. The more we practiced, the more the practice taught us, and the more we could teach others. Everywhere we went, Partner Yoga caught people's interest, and they wanted to become involved. It was the kind of practice people got excited about and were inspired to participate in. They wanted to start doing it right away. And everyone wanted a book, a manual, something they could follow when we weren't around.

Lori: *And that's just what happened. Suddenly, we weren't around. Cain went to South*

America, and I drove from Phoenix to Florida, sailed to the Bahamas, flew to Cuba and Alaska, and ended up in Colorado. We both continued to share Partner Yoga on the road, and everyone still asked, "Where's the book?" I breathed a big sigh of relief the day Cain called me from Ecuador and said, "I think I'm coming home. There's something we need to do together. Let's write that book." The wheels were rolling, and before long we were both in Hawaii writing this book.

Through the years, we continued sharing Partner Yoga with people of diverse ages, cultures, and skill levels. We carefully studied their responses and kept modifying and improving the practice. After much feedback and self-study, we have created a practice flexible enough to meet the varying needs of a diverse population. We have found that participants experience a variety of benefits. For some, Partner Yoga is simply a relaxing outlet in a busy lifestyle. Friends use it to help each other stay motivated and committed to a fitness plan. Couples find Partner Yoga to be a wonderful way to fortify trust, communication, and intimacy. Other people practice for specific health reasons. And for many, Partner Yoga is an impetus for profound spiritual growth.

Cain: *Since childhood, I have been studying various martial arts and inner disciplines, including wrestling, judo, kick boxing, yoga, Capoeira, and rock climbing (an inner discipline in its own right). Although each discipline is unique, I have never treated them as separate. My experience in each contributes something unique to the one discipline I call The Path. For me, The*

Path is characterized by a melding of diverse experiences that contribute to my physical, mental, and spiritual evolution. My work with Lori in creating Partner Yoga is largely about living this ideology to the fullest in every aspect of my life.

Lori: *Profound spiritual growth indeed! All the years of academic study, teaching, therapy, play, and colorful life experience had only begun to prepare me for this adventure. There was nowhere else to go; the journey was inside of me, and it was a blessing that My Path finally landed right next to my buddy Cain's.*

To Partner Yoga we bring 30 years of combined experience in music, medicine, dance, fitness, martial arts, and yoga. Each of these disciplines has taught us to stay keenly aware of the present moment and act creatively with a calm mind and light spirit. Above all, we've learned that life is an ocean of limitless possibilities. Practicing and teaching Partner Yoga challenges us to integrate these influences and apply everything we have learned. We continue to teach about the beauty and simplicity of mind/body wellness, the buddy system, and the importance of touch and intimacy. Partner Yoga has become our vehicle for gently taking down the walls around us and building bridges into a more harmonious world. We are developing a deeper awareness of our inner rhythms and patterns, and a sensitivity to those of others. Partner Yoga helps us to better understand ourselves and each other, and with time, it has become much more than a practice. Partner Yoga has become our way of life.

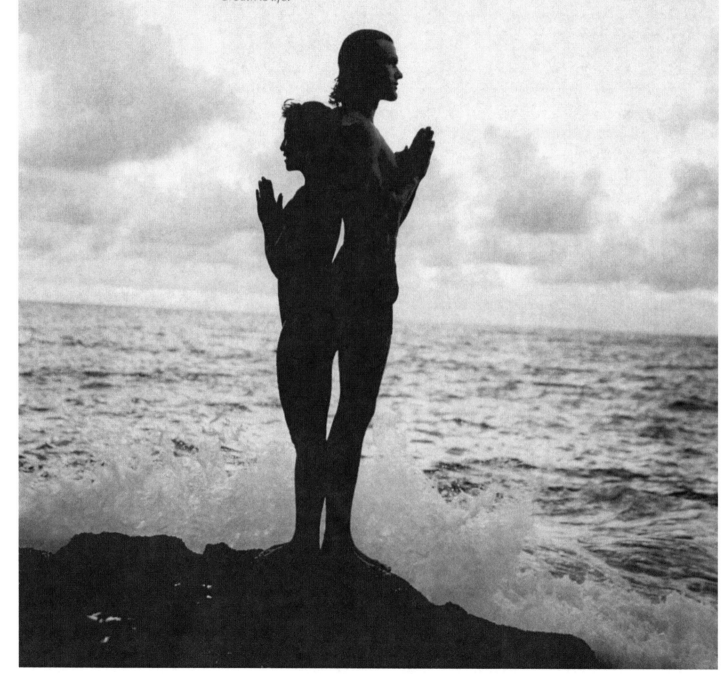

Axioms of Partner Yoga

- All things are interdependent.
- Touch and intimacy are basic human needs.
- Fear and pain are two of life's greatest teachers.
- Exercise and rest are essential for vibrant health.
- Laughter and play are life's fountains of youth.
- Partnership is based on trust and communication.
- Breath is life.

PART ONE

FOUNDATION

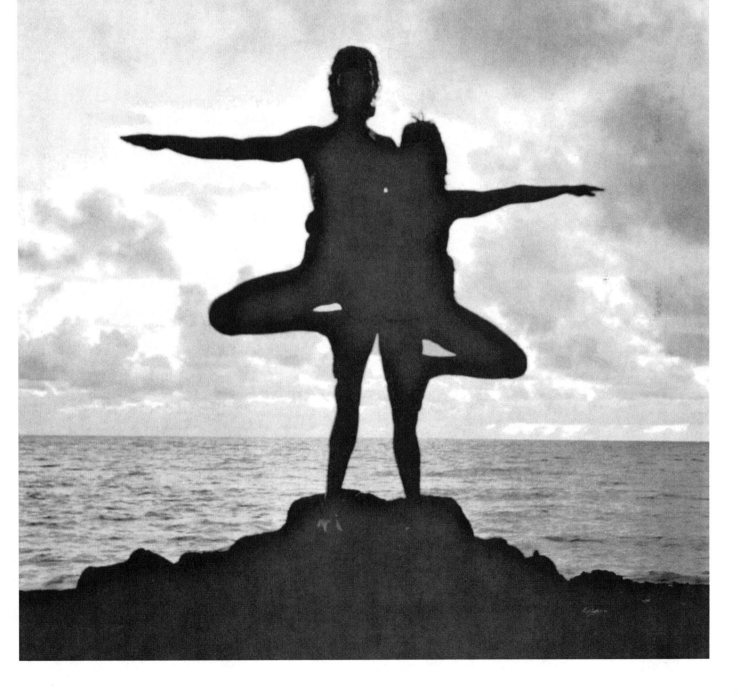

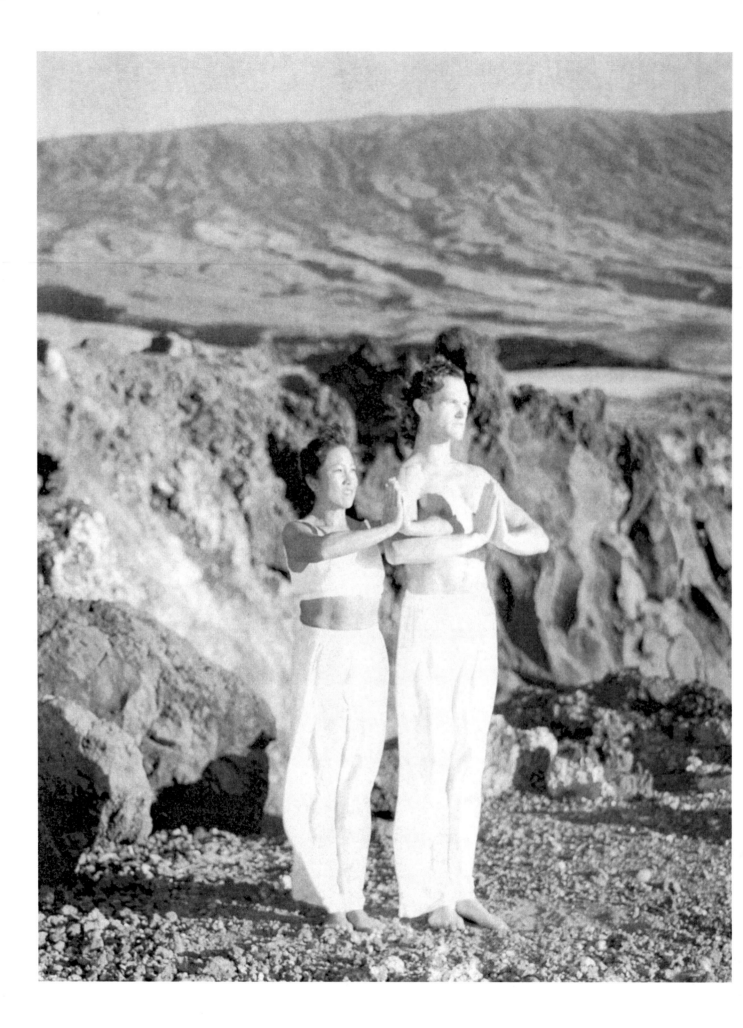

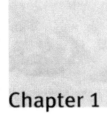

Chapter 1

Welcome to Partner Yoga

"The real voyage of discovery consists not in seeking new landscapes but in seeing with new eyes."

—Marcel Proust

Welcome. We're excited you've joined us for this journey. We've created a practice that brings two people together through yoga and touch. The practice involves physical postures, conscious breathing, touch, intimacy, trust, communication, and play. We call it Partner Yoga. Like yoga, Partner Yoga is more than just an exercise program you fit in here and there. The practice of Partner Yoga is not confined to the studio or yoga mat. Rather, this practice permeates every aspect of your life.

Partner Yoga creates the opportunity to be in an interdependent partnership. Unlike partner-assisted yoga, where one person is doing the yoga posture and another is assisting, Partner Yoga postures are mutually beneficial. For example, let's take a traditional yoga pose, or *asana*, like triangle, or *trikonasana*. You and your partner stand back to back both positioning yourselves in the triangle posture, pressing your backs into each other and linking arms as you both move into the full posture. Together you have created a new posture, which we call double triangle. This produces a completely different feeling than per-

3

forming the posture alone. Both of you are giving support and receiving benefits from the joint posture at the same time. You'll also notice that if one of you leans too much, or not enough, both of you will topple over. Exploring the perfect balance between the two of you is half the fun. The playfulness arises from the dynamic nature of partnership.

In this book, we present 60 Partner Yoga postures and three Partner Yoga flows. Some postures challenge your balance, strength, and flexibility, while others address trust and communication. Some feel so goofy you'll fall to the ground laughing, while others bring up such profound feelings they might make you cry.

When you combine your efforts and connect through touch, something magical happens. The famous psychologist Carl Jung once said, "Like any chemical reaction, when two things make contact, both are transformed."

Why Practice Partner Yoga?

Cultivating Touch

"Hands are the heart's landscape."

—Pope John Paul II

Touch transforms. All Partner Yoga postures involve touch, so we might as well

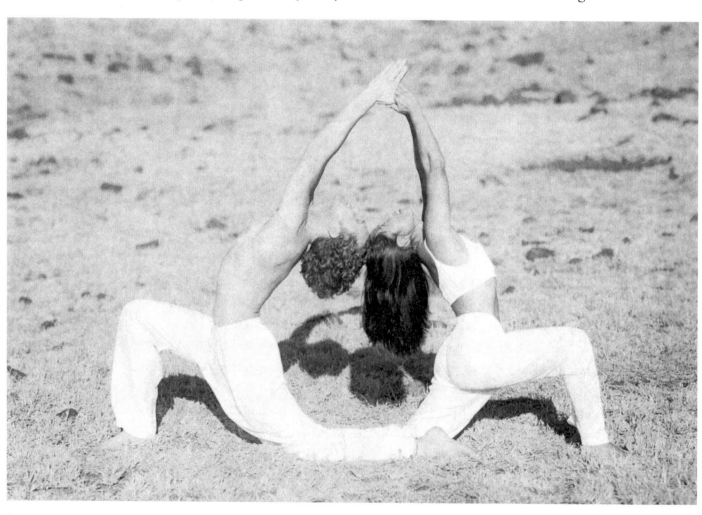

start right here. If you're going to prac-tice Partner Yoga, begin by looking at how comfortable you are with touching and being touched. Some of us are natu-rally more tactile or touch-oriented than others. This is usually a result of how we were brought up, the culture we live in, and our unique personality.

Lori: *When I was studying psychology in col-lege, I observed human behavior through field-work experiments. I would purposely touch people with my arm or leg while standing on the bus or in an elevator and would watch for reactions. I noticed how people became uncom-fortable, or apologetic, as if it were a bad thing and someone was at fault. Some people would even walk away. I noted how uptight people were about touching. When I met Cain, I learned that he still does this experiment in movie theaters and crowded elevators. It's no wonder we work so well together.*

Touch is a touchy subject. When we were babies, this didn't seem to be so. Somebody was always grooming us or wiping our bottoms. Touch was a pretty obvious necessity. In fact, scientists have learned that if an infant isn't touched, even if all other basic needs are met, that infant will suffer serious health problems.

Mary Carlson, associate professor of neuroscience in psychiatry and a science fellow at the Bunting Institute in Cambridge, Massachusetts, has spent close to 3 decades studying the effect of touch on the developing brain. Carlson

concludes that touch is crucial to the release of cortisol (an important adrenal hormone) and the regulation of our stress-response system. This influences our metabolism, immunity, and neural functioning. Children who aren't touched exhibit serious social and behavioral prob-lems such as the lack of basic emotions as well as suppressed physical growth and impaired immune systems. Studies show that these children have trouble walking, balancing, holding crayons, voicing basic needs, and remembering words.

In his ground-breaking book *Touching: The Human Significance of the Skin*, Dr. Ashley Montagu says, "Tactile needs don't change with aging. If anything, they seem to increase." Babies and infants are certainly not the only ones who need to be touched. We *all* need to touch and be touched for optimum health and happiness. Think of how nourishing skin-to-skin contact feels.

Somewhere along the way, we became wary of touching one another for fear of social, legal, or health repercussions. In the United States, we have become more accustomed to connecting with machines than connecting with our skin. Our high-tech world ties us together in many useful ways. With phones, e-mail, and television, we can link nearly every corner of the globe. Unfortunately, during the paving of these information superhighways, good old human contact got left behind. Technology is limited in its ability to truly bring us closer. A simple handshake can often tell us more about a person than the Internet or a telephone ever could.

Touch has also been misconstrued by the way our culture deals with sex. Around puberty, most people start exploring their sexual nature. Larry Dawson, in his book *Touch Not Necessarily Sex*, describes how this relationship between touch and sex became distorted in our culture. The possible implications of touch have created fear about touching. The result is a society that flip-flops between sexual overindulgence and sexual repression. We are intimacy deprived. Movies, magazine articles, lectures, and books have both contributed to and criticized this aspect of modern American culture, but no one seems to be solving the problem.

What we do know is that we are all sexual. Accepting this is the first step toward better understanding our sexual nature. Partner Yoga provides an opportunity to look at sexuality from a different angle. Physical contact may stimulate sexual feelings. Perhaps you're lying on your partner's back completely relaxed, and suddenly a sexual thought or feeling arises. Partner Yoga allows you to take a moment and simply observe what you are feeling and thinking. You don't have to repress these feelings or act on them. You can simply be with them, and in turn they will teach you more about yourself. If you jump up and run away or act immediately on these sexual feelings, you may miss a valuable opportunity. Partner Yoga is a playground for learning to embrace the various aspects of ourselves, including our sexuality.

There are many books on sacred sexuality that are specifically designed to enhance the sexual experience. Partner Yoga has a different intent. If you're practicing Partner Yoga with a sexual partner, you might still practice observing your feelings without acting on them right away. Making the conscious choice not to immediately act on your sexual inclinations provides an opportunity to experience touch and sexuality in a new way.

What would the world look like if people were more in touch with themselves and each other? How would it be different if we could let our guard down, relax, and embrace each other as our true selves? This transformation could help create a society that practices cooperation, tolerance, and interdependence. If we want to live in a more harmonious world, we could start by finding healthy ways to satisfy our basic need for touch.

Increasing Fitness

"The better you feel physically, the easier it is to be happy."

—Martin Rush

Another spoke in the health and happiness wheel depends on how fit we feel. Usually, we associate fitness with physical fitness.

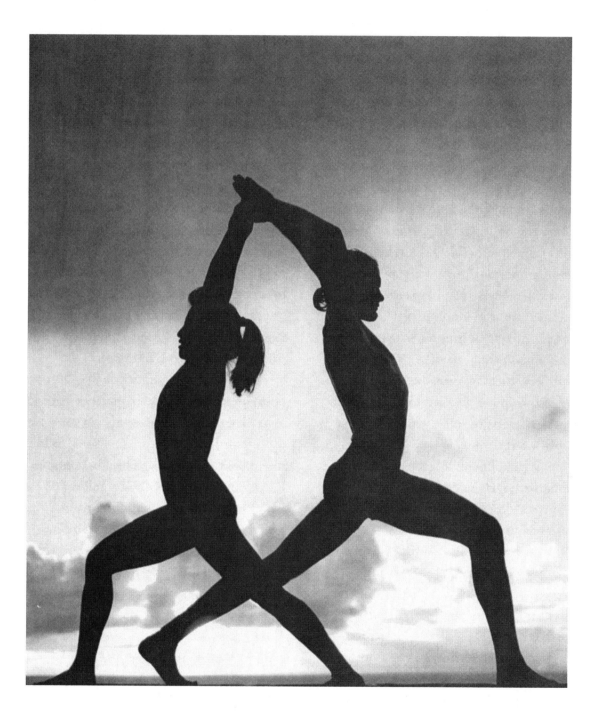

Physical fitness is certainly at the base of individual well-being. In Partner Yoga, we expand our concept of fitness to include physical, mental, emotional, and spiritual fitness. Vibrant "total-being health" is a fusion of all these aspects and more. What it means is different for everyone. Some of us are content to simply walk around the block and then curl up with a good book, while others need to do 3 hours of intense martial arts and write a software program to feel challenged. The point is that we all need to do something to stay at our optimum level of fitness.

Staying fit is a simple equation—you just need to get out there and do it. Of course, most of the time it's not that easy. Life is full of distractions. Do you ever talk yourself out of a workout because "more important" things take precedence? How often have you quit exercising because you were bored, frustrated, or just plain lazy? Getting and staying fit takes focus and motivation. Working out with a partner can make exercising more fun and help you stay on track. After all, you need to enjoy what you're doing or you'll want to quit. Postures for strength, stamina, and flexibility (see chapter 7) along with our Quick Flow and Power Flow (see chapter 10) are especially designed for fitness and fun.

Your level of physical fitness is a result of everything you do. Your job and lifestyle have as much influence on your physical fitness as your designated workout. Practicing Partner Yoga postures is a great way to support a healthy lifestyle. Breathing techniques increase lung capacity and improve circulation by working the diaphragm and back muscles. Holding physical postures develops strength and flexibility and increases the efficiency of your muscular system.

Postures that involve bending and twisting increase circulation to the spine and strengthen the entire nervous system. Twists and bends also stimulate the abdominal organs and improve digestive health. Practicing yoga builds power without rigidity and creates a supple, efficient body.

Being fit feels good. It's amazing how much more energy you have for everything when your body works efficiently. A supple body and a relaxed mind allow you to accomplish more while doing less. An important key is to keep practicing Partner Yoga with loving-kindness, patience, and a sense of humor.

Of course, sometimes you may encounter obstacles as you practice Partner Yoga. There may be moments during a posture or flow when you feel some mild discomfort and think you cannot continue. If you can breathe deeply and relax, you will release tension and gain more energy. This may enable you to do one more posture or stretch one more inch toward the ground. Each little step increases your level of fitness.

Lori: *I remember when I started running track in high school. In my first race, I thought I was going to drop dead during a 440 run. I breathed deeply, slowed to a pace where my mind stopped panicking, and somehow finished the race. By the end of the season, though, I was running cross-country without too much difficulty. The ability of*

the human body to keep stretching toward
new levels of fitness continues to amaze me.

In Partner Yoga, having a peaceful mind is the base upon which all other aspects of mental health rest. How mentally fit we are—our degree of clarity, focus, and intelligence—depends largely on how peaceful our minds are. Practicing Partner Yoga means using the entire practice—the postures, the breath, the partnership—to stop the mind from running wild.

Have you ever sat for a moment to observe what goes on in your head? For many people, that can be pretty scary. It may resemble a war zone, with thousands of thoughts and worries bombarding your mind. In Partner Yoga, you practice focusing the mind as a form of training, in order to find peace amid the chaos.

As the renowned spiritual teacher J. Krishnamurti once said, "When the mind is still, tranquil, not seeking any answer or solution, even, neither resisting nor avoiding, it is only then that there can be regeneration, because then the mind is capable of perceiving what is true and it is the truth that liberates, not our effort to be free." We practice "peaceful mind" in Partner Yoga with patience rather than force. We help each other to be good listeners. We cannot make our minds peaceful. We can only embrace our truth and allow our minds to let go of extraneous thoughts that often distract us from finding peace.

Expanding fitness to the emotional level starts with becoming more aware of what you are feeling. Your emotional fitness depends on your ability to recognize, acknowledge, and fully experience each feeling—and then to recognize its impermanence. Sometimes it's more comfortable to avoid feelings, yet they eventually catch up with you. When you suppress feelings, they become stuck and eventually begin to affect your body, mind, and spirit.

Practicing Partner Yoga can expose a wide array of feelings. When you depend on your partner for support in a lifting or leaning posture, you naturally have to trust and, to some degree, surrender. This can bring all kinds of suppressed feelings to the surface. Once again you have stumbled upon a precious opportunity for growth. If you run, fear has a hold on you. If you stay, you uncover valuable truths about yourself. In a safe arena where you feel accepted and supported, you can relax and let your feelings flow naturally. This emotional "opening" can help you feel lighter and more content.

Ultimately, as you increase your physical, mental, and emotional fitness, your spirit is happier. You've moved your body, relaxed your mind, and opened your heart. Now you can listen to your inner voice with greater clarity. Partner Yoga creates a quiet space to hear that whispering voice inside reminding you of exactly what you need to feel happy and whole.

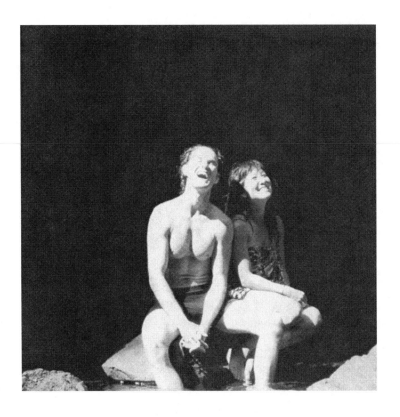

Having Fun

"The highest form of bliss is living with a certain degree of folly."

—Erasmus

Partner Yoga is meant to be playful and fun. Approach everything you do in Partner Yoga with a sense of humor and creativity. If you notice that you aren't having fun anymore, take a moment to breathe, lighten up, and ask yourself a few questions: Why am I taking this so seriously? Am I struggling to get a posture just right? Am I worried about being good enough? Am I trying to impress my partner? Sometimes we place so much importance on being "good" at things that we forget to enjoy them.

In Partner Yoga, it's not how perfectly you execute a posture, it's how much you enjoy the posture. Let's say you're moving into a posture and you're not able to stretch as far as you would like. You are disappointed and uncomfortable. You're not having fun. Here's where those "new eyes" come in. This is an opportunity to turn pain into growth, fear into courage, and resistance into acceptance. When you can redirect your self-criticism and look at yourself instead with curiosity and compassion, you have just moved a mountain. You have found a new way of being you. If you can find the ability to laugh at your shortcomings and be amused by your insecurities, life becomes less serious and more fun.

Watching children is a simple reminder of what it means to be playful and free. They have a sense of fascination and presence in whatever they do. To children, life is one big playground. As we grow older, our worries and responsibilities tend to weigh us down. When the playful child in us gets pushed aside, it affects our well-being.

Health comes with lightness and joy. In his bestseller *Anatomy of an Illness*, Norman Cousins describes how the amazing power of laughter helped to heal his own life-threatening disease.

Suffering from a serious illness and finding no success in the hospital, he decided there had to be a better way. Leaving the hospital, he checked into a hotel room where he pampered himself with funny reruns of *Candid Camera* and *The Marx Brothers*. Laughter turned out to be a potent medicine. Experiencing joy and laughter on a regular basis can significantly affect our lives. Mr. Cousins regained his health and went on to write and lecture about how affirmative emotions affect body chemistry, and how important they are for our lives. As you practice Partner Yoga, remember this story and encourage your inner child to come out and play. Find things to laugh about. Allow yourself to be silly and spontaneous, even goofy.

Relaxing

"Practice not-doing, and everything will fall into place."

—Tao Te Ching

Many of you are exploring Partner Yoga for contact, fitness, or fun. Some of you just want to chill. Either way, we'd prefer that Partner Yoga doesn't end up as another item on your "to do" list. Most of you already have enough to do. In fact, our culture places so much importance on what we do that we are starting to

become a race of human "doings" instead of human beings. Partner Yoga is about learning to relax and "just be." Rushing to do postures is like speeding to a massage appointment and then running off to the next activity—you hardly get to taste the sweetness of what you're experiencing. If you catch yourself thinking of relaxation as something that has to be done, you're missing the point. Relaxation is a state of being. Dr. Deepak Chopra said it well in a lecture: "It is when we slip into the gaps of being that we find wholeness."

As you practice Partner Yoga, take some time to look at how you are managing the stressors in your life. For many of us, stress and tension are such a normal part of our lives that we sometimes aren't even aware they're there. Having stress is usually not the problem, however; stress is simply another experience. It's how we manage the stress that causes the problem.

Remember to help your partner stay aware of how she holds tension. Sometimes she may not even realize that her shoulders are tense. As you practice partner postures, stay relaxed in your shoulders and hands, which are two good indicators of tension. It may seem like gripping your partner's hand in certain postures makes the posture more secure. Most of the time, though, that's not the case. With practice, you realize that holding your partner's hand in a firm yet relaxed way is much more effective.

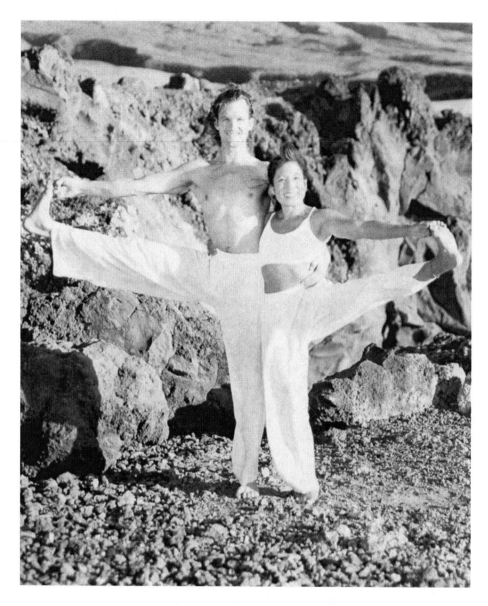

me to be in his wedding in California. On the way back to Hawaii, I got stuck for 7 hours at the international airport and decided to turn the unfortunate change of plans into a field study on relationships. I wandered around the airport asking people of diverse ages and ethnicities to share their recipes for a successful relationship. Although the people's accents and skin colors varied greatly, their responses were surprisingly similar. Every person I asked mentioned communication as one of the main ingredients of a good relationship.

Our conversations are a reflection of our everyday experiences and the events of our time. Maybe that's why people are always talking about relationships and the weather; the two are timeless topics that affect every aspect of our lives. Think for a moment about the vast matrix of relationships that make up your environment. The most obvious ones are your relationships with friends, family, and coworkers. How about your relationship to pets, plants, your home, the weather, and our planet? Finally, how do you relate to yourself?

The last question is the one we are most interested in. How do you commu-

Strengthening Relationships

"Without relationship, there is no existence: To be is to be related."

—J. Krishnamurti, renowned spiritual teacher

Cain: *I was in the middle of working on this section about relationships when a friend asked*

nicate with yourself? Are you kind? Are you tactful? Do you accept yourself? Do you respect yourself? Do you trust yourself? Do you enjoy your own company? Do you like yourself? Do you love yourself?

It may seem silly to answer these questions, yet the responses will unveil the foundation upon which all of your other relationships are built. There are no right answers, and nobody is waiting for a response. So take a little time to digest these questions. Respond to yourself honestly, without regard for how you "should" feel or what your response "ought" to be.

Because of our busy lifestyles, we don't take much time to cultivate a relationship with ourselves. When we do, we usually feel more grounded and centered. In our relationships with other people, we are required to fill many roles—teachers, students, parents, lovers, professionals—and it's easy to get pulled off center. In dance or the martial arts, for example, you learn to move *from* your center without being pulled off it. Your center is the source of your balance, power, and truth; to abandon your center in dance or the martial arts is virtually a sin. In our daily relationships, the same principle applies. In relationships, "moving from your center" means having a deeper understanding of who you are; it means first establishing an honest relationship within yourself and then sharing that person with others. Of course, being real with ourselves can be a humbling or

even frightening experience. There are parts of ourselves we would rather ignore, let alone share with others. So we become masters of illusion. With shades of truth, we paint a personality we can accept and, in turn, present to the world. Some of us have created such a masterpiece that even we cannot remember who we really are.

Building a strong center begins with acceptance of the real you, the whole you—even the parts you don't like. If you can approach this relationship with yourself with a sense of intrigue, humor, and compassion, all of your other relationships will follow suit. There are no magic methods or shortcuts. Yogi J. Krishnamurti puts it best when he writes, "There is no path to truth. Truth must be discovered, but there is no formula for its discovery. What is formulated is not true. You must set out on the uncharted sea, and the uncharted sea is yourself."

Most of you will choose a Partner Yoga partner with whom you have an established relationship. That person may be a fitness buddy, your child, or your lover. The physical contact, communication, and mutual support required to practice Partner Yoga can certainly strengthen that relationship. In the case of a fitness buddy, for example, you are building trust and serving as mirrors for each other as you help each other with alignment, balance, and concentration. Each of you learns more about yourself with the help of your buddy.

Partner Yoga uses the good old buddy system that has been around for ages. Tested through time, we know the buddy system works. Looking out for each other, finding safety in pairs, and watching your partner's back are familiar concepts to most of us. As kids, we were taught to hold hands when crossing the street and to always travel with a buddy. As we get older, many activities use this same concept. Scuba diving, weight lifting, and rock climbing, for example, use the buddy system for safety and support. Partner Yoga postures use the buddy system in similar ways. If you notice that your partner is stepping way out of alignment in a posture or that his attention seems to be waning, you can encourage him back. At other times, you will be physically supporting your partner and literally watching out for his safety. Partner postures remind us of how important it is to have a buddy and what it really means to be one.

If you have chosen to practice Partner Yoga with your child, you are bound to have some fun and to get to know each other in a whole new way. Children sometimes have idealized concepts of their parents: Parents are always right; they are always strong; and parents know everything. Of course, we all know none of these claims are true (although parents may not want to hear that). If you practice Partner Yoga with your child, make him or her feel like your

equal, your buddy, your partner. Approach the activity with an added element of honesty and vulnerability, and your relationship will certainly deepen.

If you practice Partner Yoga with your lover, you have a great opportunity to further your intimacy. Listen to the sound of each other's breath and synchronize your breathing patterns. Together move slowly through poses with grace and sensitivity. Stay acutely aware of each other's physical structure and alignment. Practice trusting each other to the extent that you feel almost uncomfortable. And occasionally, with mindful courage, attempt a pose or variation that takes you both to your edge.

What Do *You* Need?

Sometimes asking for what you need isn't easy. We've been conditioned to hide our feelings and our needs. In our culture, asking for what we need is often seen as a sign of weakness. In Partner Yoga, expressing your needs is a sign of strength. If we could read each other's minds and fill each other's needs without having to ask, that would be different. The truth is that this rarely happens, and asking for what we need is necessary. Can you step out of your old habits and create new ways of being?

A great yogi once said, "If you want to create a new body, then step out of the river of conditioning and see the world as if for the first time—use memory but do not allow memory to use you—step out of the river and look at an ordinary object through the eyes of innocence, not through the camouflage of your labels and definitions and descriptions and evaluations and analysis."

A willingness to ask for what you need as well as to support those around you may take a shift in conditioning or perspective. There is a story about a farmer who grew award-winning corn. A newspaper reporter asked him how he did it, and the farmer told him that when his neighbors asked, he shared his prize seed corn with them. Surprised, the reporter asked him how he could afford to share his best seed with his neighbors when they were all entering corn in the same competition. The farmer answered, "Why sir, didn't you know? The wind picks up pollen from the ripening corn and swirls it from field to field. If my neighbors grow inferior corn, cross-pollination will steadily degrade the quality of my corn. If I am to grow good corn, I must help my neighbors to grow good corn."

So it is with happiness. If we want to be happy or be at peace, we must support our neighbors in being happy or being at peace. The wellness of each person is affected by the wellness of all. The value of our lives is a reflection of the lives we touch. If we want to cultivate our inner joy and wisdom, we need to help others cultivate theirs. And only by helping each other can we create unity. This is the Partner Yoga principle.

The Territory Is Yours to Discover

Through the process of our own exploration of Partner Yoga and the experience of coauthoring this book, we have confronted all of the issues discussed here together, as partners. To be honest, it was not easy and we did not always agree. Yet we stayed committed to finding ways to make it work. Along the road there were no footsteps to follow and no magic solutions. The answers came when we spent less time searching outside of ourselves and more time looking within. Each day of our lives, we are confronted with this challenge. As you embark upon your own experience in Partner Yoga, we ask that you do what feels true for you. We ask that you honestly communicate with your partner. And most important, we ask that you take the experience inward and remind your partner to do the same.

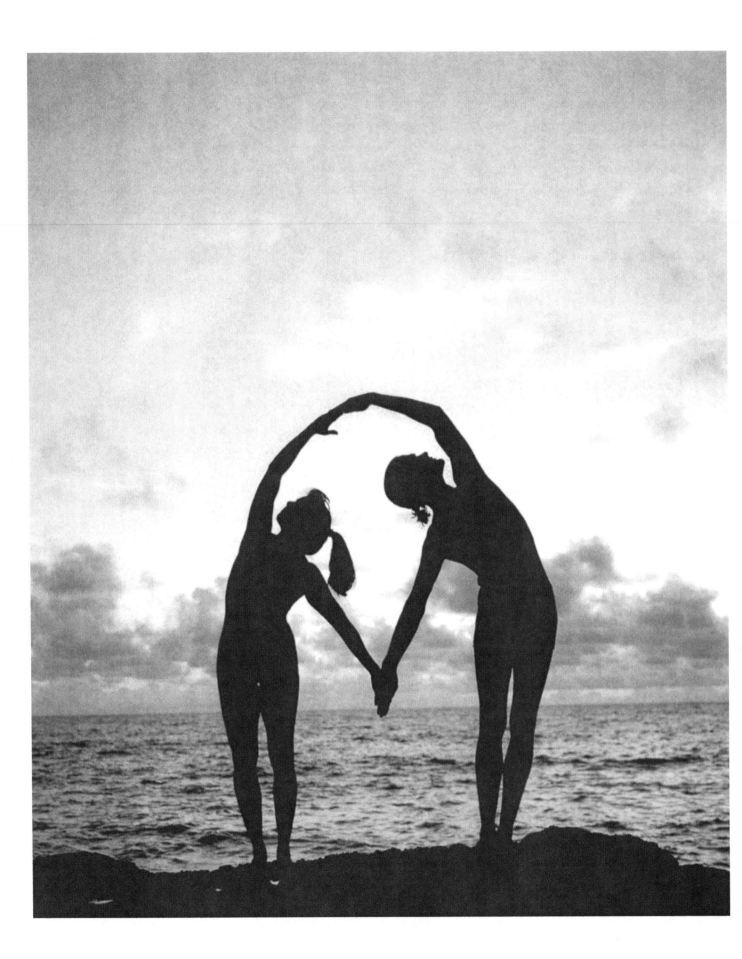

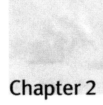

Chapter 2

Building on a Timeless Tradition

"Growing is the most important and essential endeavor that a human being can undertake."

—Swami Chetananda

Now that you understand the fundamentals of Partner Yoga, let's look at this new discipline in context of the larger tradition of yoga. The word "yoga" comes from the Sanskrit root *yug*, meaning to attach, join, yoke, or connect. Yoga can also mean "to attain what was previously unattainable," or "to cause change." For example, consider the example of the farmer who has both an ox and a plow but no way to join the two. Alone neither can create the desired change. Only after the yoke is placed on the ox and the plow is connected can the farmer begin to till his soil. In this case, it is the joining, or yoga, of the ox and plow that enables the farmer to attain something that was previously unattainable. The teachings of yoga would refer to the joining of ox and plow as much more than just a connection. Rather, this relationship is refered to as "union." In essence, the word yoga connotes a mystical state of union between forces of energy.

The practice of Partner Yoga is much like the scenario of the farmer. By simply finding a partner and agreeing to practice a few postures, you are already experiencing yoga. In this case, you have made a connection that will inevitably cause change. Perhaps after a short session, you can breathe easier, you feel taller, or you're just more relaxed. The mere fact that you noticed a shift in your breathing implies that you have made another important connection—this time between your body and mind. In yoga, it is said that breathing is what links the body and mind. Simply put, breathing is yoga.

When your breathing is smooth, your mind is calm and your body becomes free of tension. In Partner Yoga, we use con-scious breathing to create awareness of how the various aspects of our bodies and minds interact and how we interact with our partners. When all of these aspects are in harmony, there is a sense of wholeness and a feeling of connection. This leads toward the ultimate goal of yoga, a state of inner joy and outer unity.

The Roots

To get a clearer view of what yoga is and where it can take you, let's take a look at its mysterious history. Among teachers and

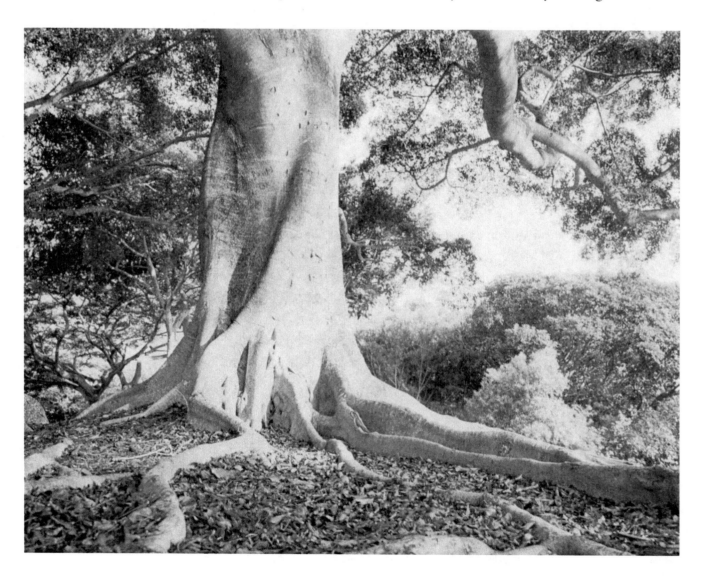

students, it is commonly believed that the practice of yoga is more than 5,000 years old. Historically, the teachings of yoga were passed orally from teacher to student, often with little or no textual documentation, making it difficult to ascertain the exact age of yoga.

What we do know is that yoga originated in India as one of the six orthodox systems of philosophy collectively known as *darshana*. As one of the *darshana*, the teachings of yoga are deeply rooted in Vedic scriptures, the oldest and most venerated record of Indian culture. Since yoga evolved in the context of Hinduism, it is imbued with the flavor of Hindu symbols and mythology. Many yoga postures are named after Hindu gods or mythological heroes. However, yoga is not a religion. Yoga is an art and a science. In yoga, emphasis is placed on experimentation and personal discovery. Even though yoga is associated with certain traditions and

metaphysical notions, the practice of yoga does not ask you to believe in anything you have not experienced yourself. In fact, the only prerequisite for practicing yoga is a desire for growth and a spirit for adventure.

The Ancient Yogis Were Just like You

Like many of us, the forefathers of yoga were explorers in search of the secrets of a healthy, happy life. These sages did not set out to put themselves in pretzel poses. Rather, they were fueled by the idea that life has something deeper and more meaningful to offer. While sitting for hours in meditation, the sages quickly realized that exploration is not easy—particularly on the knees and ankles—and that a strong, supple body and sharp mental focus would be necessary to make the journey. The complex system of exercises and stretches we now call *hatha yoga* was born from this need. All the stretching and moving you now do in yoga was originally designed to help you sit still and focus your attention inward.

Through the centuries, yogis looked within themselves to find the answers to life's questions. They explored new territory and experimented with new techniques; most important, they passed their discoveries on to others. Around the 2nd century CE (Common Era), an Indian sage named Patanjali systematized and recorded

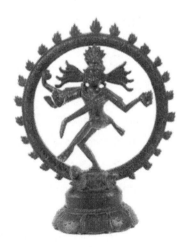

the developing science of yoga in the famous *Yoga Sutra*, often referred to as the heart of yoga. The *Yoga Sutra* is composed of 195 aphorisms that lay the foundation for a deep and meaningful practice of yoga. Above all, the *Yoga Sutra* addresses the subtle issues of the human mind, moral integrity, and inner stillness. It alludes to the ultimate goal of yoga as unity of body, mind, and spirit, and a mystical connection to something larger, a connection to all Creation.

Interestingly, the *Yoga Sutra* mentions no physical yoga poses other than the seated meditation posture. Not until centuries later would a text be written about the physical aspects of yoga. Even then, such classical texts as the *Hatha Yoga Pradipika* (written in the 14th century) and the *Gheranda Samhita* (written in the 17th century) only make reference to a handful of physical postures. In the yoga community, legends tell of other influential texts, such as the *Yoga Korunta* (allegedly inscribed on palm leaves) and the *Yoga*

Rahasya, that are said to have been lost or destroyed over time.

In the mid-1980s, a yoga scholar named Norman Sjoman made a discovery that would shed new light on the obscure history of yoga. While doing research in the private library of the Maharaja of Mysore (at the Mysore Palace in India), Sjoman happened upon a yoga manual from the 1800s called the *Sritattvanidhi*. The *Sritattvanidhi* contains elaborate instructions for and illustrations of 122 physical yoga postures—making it the most detailed text on the yoga postures written before the 20th century. Reportedly, the text is written by a Mysore prince of the same royal family that would, a century later, join forces with the modern yoga master T. Krishnamachariya and his world-famous students, B.K.S. Iyengar and Pattabhi Jois (respectively, the originators of Iyengar Yoga and Ashtanga Yoga, two of today's most commonly practiced styles of yoga).

Yoga made its way to the United States in 1893 when Swami Vivekananda, a dis-

Language of the Gods

Many of the words we use in yoga, such as asana *(pose) or* prana *(life force), come from ancient texts written in Sanskrit. Oftentimes these words represent ideas and principles that do not easily translate to English or other Western languages. Although the exact age of Sanskrit is still uncertain, scholars speculate that Sanskrit may in fact be one of the world's oldest languages. Among sages and mystics, Sanskrit is considered sacred, and it is believed that the spoken word is imbued with spiritual qualities. Sanskrit is called Devanagari, the language of the gods, and many people believe that speaking or chanting in Sanskrit opens the door to higher consciousness.*

ciple of the highly venerated Indian sage Ramakrishna, arrived at the World Fair in Chicago to present a talk on the philosophy of yoga. This auspicious meeting of East and West denotes the inception of the American yoga movement. By the early 1900s, yoga centers were popping up in numerous U.S. cities and several other Indian yogis had already landed on American soil—among them Paramahansa Yogananda, author of the world-renowned *Autobiography of a Yogi*.

Yoga in the Era of Endless Possibilities

There have always been countless ways to practice yoga, and you can behold this generation's incarnations by visiting any one of the growing number of yoga centers throughout the world. From Karma Yoga (the practice of yoga as service) to Power Yoga (an intense physical practice), there exists an almost overwhelming gamut of practices called "yoga." One school offers spiritual enlightenment, while another shows you how to put your foot behind your head. The fitness industry is hot on yoga. Celebrities are practicing yoga. Doctors are recommending yoga for their patients. Outwardly, yoga is taking many shapes. Western culture has embraced yoga, and the possibilities are endless. As the limelight shines on yoga, however, it yields mixed messages. We see yogis in car ads, Hindu gods on mini skirts, and flashes of yoga in the popular media. While the hype surrounding yoga can be exciting, the use of these images may be misleading.

It comes as no surprise that as yoga enters the mainstream, it becomes adorned with ornaments of our material culture. Unlike their predecessors, modern yogis now wear spandex and nail polish and practice postures on thin purple mats. Yet, loincloth or leotard, yogis are united by a common thread that transcends time and culture. In presenting this practice of Partner Yoga, our foremost intention is to honor this thread by continuing to do what yogis have done since time immemorial—look deep within ourselves, experiment, innovate, and share what we've learned with others.

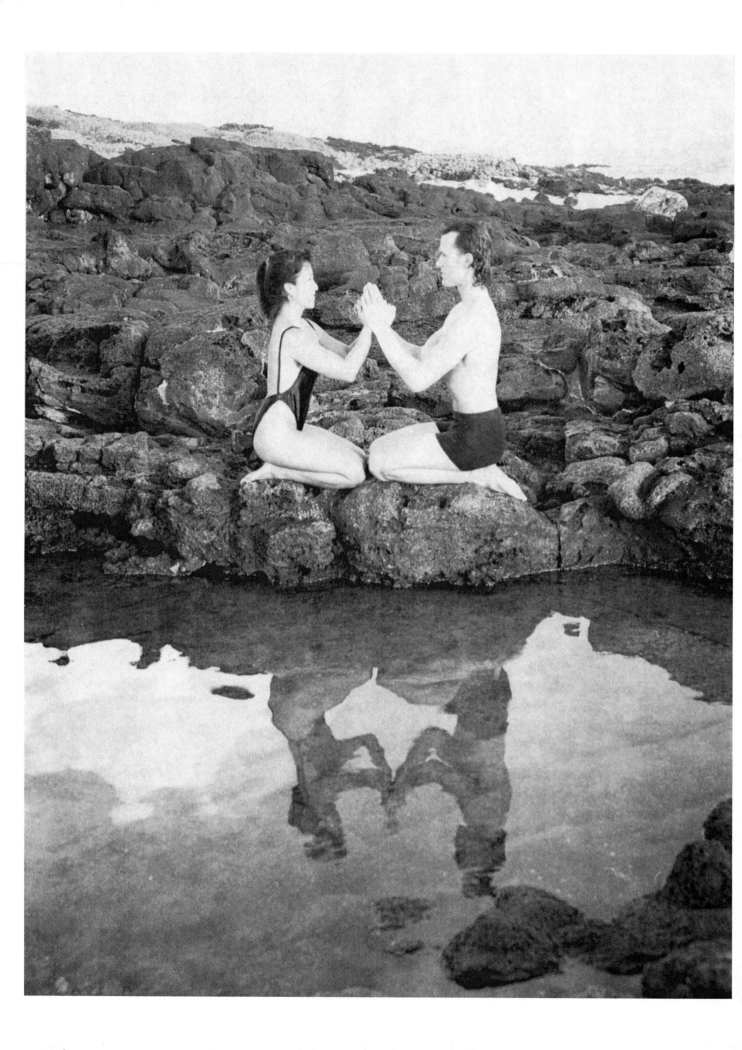

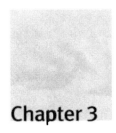

Chapter 3

Making Contact

"A simple, divine smile may change more hearts than a thousand windy sermons or learned treatises."

—Swami Kriyananda

As you embark on your Partner Yoga adventure, take a moment to make sure you have everything you need. If you were going on a camping trip, you would want to know what to take and how best to prepare. Let's look at the practical essentials for starting Partner Yoga.

People come to Partner Yoga for a variety of reasons—longing for a new experience, expanding an existing yoga practice, desiring physical contact, fitness, fun, relaxation, or intimacy. Being clear about your intentions can help you make choices about the practical aspects of Partner Yoga, like whom you choose as a partner and where, when, and how you practice. If you just want to practice and you're not sure why, simply find a person who is interested in practicing with you and see what unfolds. Ultimately, your experience will take on its own unique form. When you truly make contact, miracles happen.

Partnering Up

Newcomers to Partner Yoga might think that it is primarily for couples. We want to re-emphasize the fact that Partner Yoga is for everyone. If you are in a primary relationship, practicing Partner Yoga together can deepen your relationship. You can also benefit from practicing Partner Yoga with people other than your primary partner. If this brings up intimacy issues, peek ahead to chapter 14.

There are many creative options in partnering. Is there someone you would like to get to know better or spend a little time with? Is there someone at the gym you think would make a good fitness buddy? Do you have a friend you enjoy being with yet rarely get to see? Would you like to spend more time doing something fun and creative with your primary partner? When choosing a partner, ask yourself if you could relax with this person, or at least be willing to learn how to relax with them. If you are practicing Partner Yoga mainly to relieve tension, consider your lover, housemate, or a friend. If you are practicing Partner Yoga for fitness, a coworker or gym buddy might work out well.

On Location

After you have found someone to practice with, the next question is the location. If you're practicing the Quick Flow with someone (see chapter 10) or throwing together a few partner postures for a quick stretch in between other activities, you can pretty much practice anywhere. If you want to practice for a longer period of time or explore either the fitness or relax-

ation flows, choosing an appropriate space is essential.

The basic necessities for your practice space are pretty simple: flat, safe, comfortable, and quiet. In other words, somewhere you can relax. If there are swarming mosquitoes, loud construction noise, and a hill you keep sliding down, it's not going to work. If your intent is to relax, practicing outdoors is fine as long as you're not in the hot sun, freezing cold, or wind. The home is a nice place to be intimate, relax, and unwind. If you're practicing for fitness, the gym, your home, or a park works well.

Depending on the space you choose, a mat or blanket might be necessary for padding. A rug, blanket, yoga mat, or large beach towel is good as long as it isn't too slippery for standing postures. Practicing Partner Yoga directly on the earth is a grounding experience and works well for many of the postures. With so many options, you have an opportunity to create an environment that satisfies your needs.

Time Keeps On Ticking

"You will never 'find' time for anything. If you want time, you must make it."

—Charles Buxton

So you have the "what," the "who," and the "where." Now the clincher is when. Some of you have lots of free time, and some of you are praying for the clock to slow down long enough for you to catch up. Either way, you need to set a specific time to practice Partner Yoga or it probably won't happen. We've all said those famous last words: "That looks like fun, let's do it sometime." Even if we know we would enjoy the activity, somehow "sometime" never comes. When time schedules get tight, essential needs and desires demand our attention. The truth is that exercise, relaxation, emotional support, and intimacy are all essential.

If you and your yoga partner live together or close by, you might consider practicing Partner Yoga in the mornings or before bed. Be creative and realistic. You probably will not continue practicing if you have to drive long distances or wake up at an unreasonable hour to meet your partner. If you make the practice fit into your life as easily as possible, it is more likely to become an ongoing practice.

Contact Questions

You have the basics and are ready to begin. Do you still have a few questions? This section addresses some of the subtle details of making contact.

Q. What is the ideal amount of time to set aside for practicing Partner Yoga?
A. If you want to do more than a couple of quick stretches, set aside at least 30 min-

utes to practice. An hour to an hour and a half is probably more ideal. If you can allow more time, spend as much time as your heart desires.

Q. What is the best time of day to practice?
A. Practicing Partner Yoga in the morning is like a strong cup of coffee without the side effects. Most of us are a little stiff and groggy in the morning, and a gentle stretch can get the blood flowing and jump-start our day. Partner Yoga in the afternoon or evening can help relieve the tension of the day, calm the mind, and bring you back to balance for a peaceful night of sleep.

Q. How long do you recommend holding postures?
A. If you are practicing for fitness, it is best to move through postures a little quicker to elevate your heart rate. If you're unwinding after a long day or nudging your body to get up in the morning, move into postures slowly and hold them longer. (At the beginning, you may be able to hold only for a few seconds; eventually, you will be able to hold for 30 seconds to a minute or up to 5 minutes for some of the more relaxing postures.) You don't ever want to hold a posture so long that you feel dizzy or faint. Remember that moving in and out of postures with control is as important as completing the finished pose.

Q. Do I need to bring anything else besides this book to my first Partner Yoga session?

A. If you want to practice synchronized breathing (see page 33) or meditation, a small pillow to lift your buttocks off the ground is useful. Wear appropriate clothes for the weather so you won't be chilled when sitting quietly. Bring a mat or blanket depending on your practice space. Other than that, you're set. All you really need is a creative mind, a courageous spirit, and an open heart.

Q. Do I need to find a partner with the same level of yoga experience as I have?

A. Beginners and advanced yogis can both benefit from Partner Yoga practice. Naturally, two advanced yogis can explore more challenging postures. If you are more advanced and choose to practice with a beginner, you can polish up on basic alignment and have an opportunity to practice patience. Seeing yoga from a beginner's viewpoint can give you a new perspective. There is much we can learn from each other if we take the time and embrace the lessons.

Q. Do my partner and I need to be the same height and weight?

A. There are advantages and disadvantages to having a partner of similar size. It is often easier to practice with someone of a similar size. Having a partner who is a different size than you, however, can stimulate creativity and lead to creative posture

variations that accommodate the differences. Learning to adjust your postures around these variables can be an interesting adventure.

Q. Is it best to partner with someone whose flexibility and fitness level is the same as mine?

A. Varying levels of flexibility are not a major concern. You will both benefit from Partner Yoga regardless of how flexible you are. For the most part, the same is true of fitness. If you are practicing specifically to get in shape, however, it is best to find a partner who is in similar physical condition.

Q. What if one of us is not feeling well, is injured, or has a specific health concern? Should we still practice Partner Yoga?

A. As long as your approach is conscious, Partner Yoga can be helpful when you are injured, ill, or have a specific health concern. Once again, communication is key. Refer to chapter 11 for specific posture ideas. Also refer to the Benefits and Cautions sections for the individual postures.

Q. What if my partner or I have issues around touching or intimacy? Does Partner Yoga have to be intimate?

A. Partner Yoga is whatever you make of it. The practice can be as casual as two buddies jogging or as intimate as two souls communing. Physical contact can be explored in many different ways. Keep the channels of communication clear and move into uncomfortable territory with an open mind. Chapter 14 goes into this subject in more detail.

Q. I'm concerned about issues of jealousy that might arise if I practice Partner Yoga with someone other than my sexual partner. Any suggestions?

A. Be genuine with yourself and your partner from the beginning. If you want to practice yoga with someone other than your primary partner, be clear about your intent. Maybe you want to practice with a coworker during lunch on Tuesday and a gym buddy after work on Thursday. Can your sexual partner be comfortable with that? People put expectations and limitations on each other all the time. Fear and jealousy pose challenges in many relationships. Openly addressing these feelings with courage and honesty can strengthen the relationship. One of the intentions of Partner Yoga is to widen our views of partnership and intimacy, which is explored in chapter 14.

Q. Is Partner Yoga the same as Tantric yoga?

A. No, the focus of Partner Yoga is not sexual. In fact, contrary to popular belief, not all Tantric yoga is sexual. Partner Yoga does, however, embrace many of the same principles as Tantric yoga. Partner Yoga can be practiced by any two people: friends, coworkers, parents and kids, or lovers. The intent of Partner Yoga is to bring people together through movement, play, breath, touch, and intimacy. Partner Yoga, like Tantric yoga, acknowledges and honors the power of two people to transcend limitations, strengthen relationships, and ultimately feel a deep sense of connection to the Divine.

Q. I have a difficult time focusing inward when I practice yoga alone. Will practicing with a partner help this, or could it distract me more?

A. Practicing yoga with a partner actually helps you direct your attention inward. As buddies, you serve as mirrors for each other and help each other stay on track. Most important, you help each other bridge your inner truths with your outward actions. As we've said before, Partner Yoga is ultimately a journey to your true self.

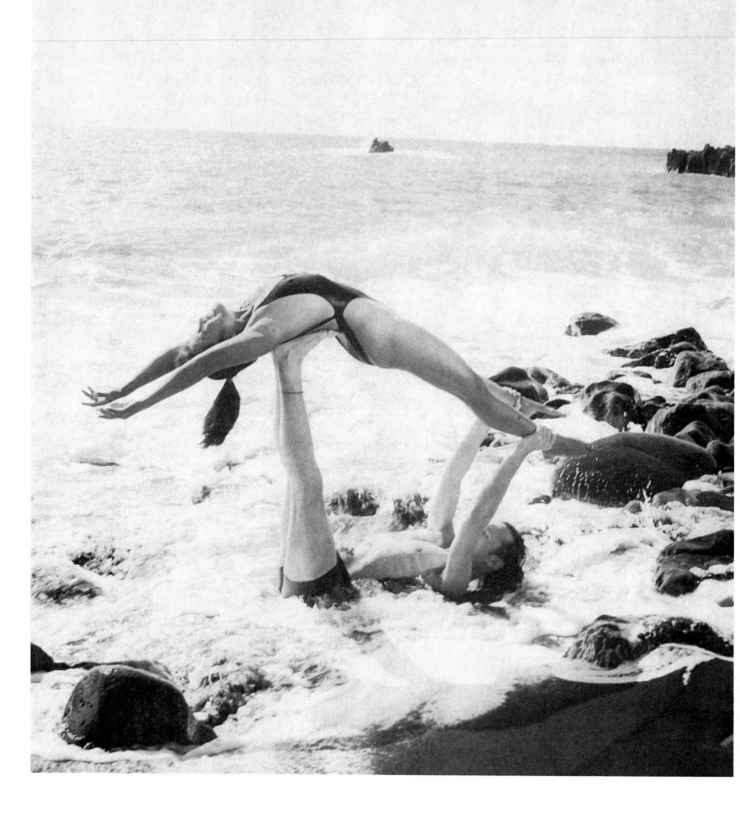

Chapter 4

Breath Is Life

"Yogis count life not by number of years but number of breaths."

—Swami Vishnudevananda

As modern-day yogis, our challenges are very different than those of our Indian predecessors. The modern world is overwhelmingly complex, featuring full schedules and overflowing "to do" lists. Meeting the demands of everyday life requires focus, organization, and resourcefulness. Somewhere between our daily planner and our e-mail inbox, we often lose sight of the importance of satisfying our most basic human need, breathing. On average, we breathe about 23,000 times a day, which amounts to about 4,500 gallons of air. Yet the *quality* of our breathing is often lacking.

Let's compare breathing with eating. We breathe and eat to stay alive. We have become aware that the quality of what we eat is as important as eating itself. The same is true of breathing. The quality of each breath we take largely determines how we feel and function. In a sense, breathing is part of our nutrition program.

While the saying "you are what you eat" might seem trite, what you put into your body does directly affect how your body functions. This principle is not limited to food, however. It includes everything you take in: liquids, smells, sights, sounds, touch, and, of course, breath. Since breathing plays a vital role in everything else you do, it might be more accurate to say, "You are your breath." Better breathing fills you with nourishment. It is at the center of all human life.

Breathe like Babies Do

In yoga, breath is called *prana*, which means life, vitality, or strength. Yoga texts refer to *prana* as the universal life force, "a vibrant psychophysical energy similar to the *pneuma* of the ancient Greeks." Indeed, breathing is the first thing we do when we come into the world, and it's the last thing we do when we leave. Every moment in between is connected by breath. As infants and toddlers, we were masters of the fine art of effective breathing. Our bodies were supple and free of tension. We maximized our intake of air by expanding through the chest, back, ribs, and abdomen. Our breathing was dynamic and we bubbled with boundless energy.

As we grew older, the pressures of young adulthood began to close in on us like a boa constrictor. Girls were told to "suck it in" and boys learned to "suck it up." Each year, the demands of our peers, parents, and culture increased. By the time we graduated to "maturity," we had learned to harden ourselves to avoid collapsing under the weight of it all.

As adults, we are continually burdened with anxiety and tension. Many of us have lost touch with what we instinctively knew at birth. As responsibilities pile up, our chests and shoulders tighten and our breathing becomes shallow. When we get excited or agitated, we clench our stomach muscles and tighten our necks. Many of us live in a constant state of contraction, which robs us of free-flowing energy and constricts the flow of oxygen to our brains and the rest of our bodies. Unfortunately, our culture regards the

Quality Control

Here are some simple suggestions for "high quality" breathing.

- *Breathe through your nose; the nostrils are nature's air filter and conditioner.*
- *Relax your shoulders, chest, ribs, and abdomen, and allow your diaphragm to do its job. Breathing diaphragmatically naturally massages the abdominal organs.*
- *Allow your inhalations to become smooth and deep, and your exhalations to be long and complete.*
- *Learn to feel your breath in the sides and back of your body.*
- *Make breathing a mindful practice. Post "Remember to Breathe" notes in your car, in your daily planner, at your desk, and on the fridge.*
- *Remind your partner to practice all of the above.*

repercussions—fatigue, headaches, high blood pressure, neck and back pain—as merely part of life. Modern medicine offers some quick fixes, yet it usually neglects to address the root cause.

In many ways, Partner Yoga serves to reconnect you with the building blocks of life. As you practice the partner postures, immerse yourself in the raw experience of movement, touch, and play. Allow yourself to feel uninhibited and perhaps a little vulnerable. Increasing the level of basic expression helps you reintegrate a part of yourself that remembers how to live lightly and how to breathe. In *The Breathing Book*, author Donna Farhi refers to this unconditioned breath as the "essential breath," or "the breath you breathed as a young child." As Farhi asserts, "Opening the door to this life force involves rediscovering the virgin nature of the breath."

Show Me Yours and I'll Show You Mine

Understanding the basics of breathing anatomy can promote breath awareness. Don't worry, we won't ask you to memorize the entire respiratory system, nor will there be a multiple choice test later. Rather, we ask you and your partner to *experience* the various parts of your own breathing anatomy and become familiar with how they function.

The process of respiration originates at the cellular level. Every cell in the body needs oxygen. Breathing is our response to this need. To begin the process of satisfying our cells, we draw air into our lungs by engaging an amazing system of muscles that work to create a vacuum. The primary muscles used in breathing are the diaphragm, the intercostal muscles, and the abdominal muscles. There are also numerous secondary, or accessory, muscles that aid the process of breathing (especially during exercise or vigorous activity). Among them are the scalenus, sternocleidomastoid, pectoralis, trapezius, latissimus dorsi, serratus anterior and posterior, rhomboideus minor and major, and the internal and external oblique muscles. Although each of these muscles contributes to the breathing process, the diaphragm is responsible for 70 to 80 percent of the normal workload.

The diaphragm is a huge dome-shaped muscle that separates the chest cavity from the abdomen. Above the diaphragm sit the heart and lungs (the heart actually rides on top of the diaphragm, connected by a smooth connective tissue called fascia). Below the diaphragm are the abdominal organs that perform digestion, assimilation, and elimination. To draw air into the lungs, the diaphragm contracts and presses downward against these organs and expands the ribs up and out (laterally). Consequently, the volume of the lungs increases and, by nature of the vacuum, air rushes in to fill the space. The process of breathing is less an act of "taking in" air and more an act of providing an open space for the breath to fill.

The Explorations

To help launch the journey back to your essential breath, perform the following explorations with your partner.

Exploration I—Feeling the Breath

Is your breathing shallow or deep? Rapid or slow? This exploration is designed to help you become aware of your breathing. Sit facing your partner in a comfortable position. You may want to sit on the floor in a cross-legged position or in a chair. If you choose to sit in a chair, sit toward the front edge, with your feet flat on the ground and your spine erect.

Close your eyes and begin "observing" your breath. Simply relax, and let yourself breathe naturally without intentionally altering your breath or performing

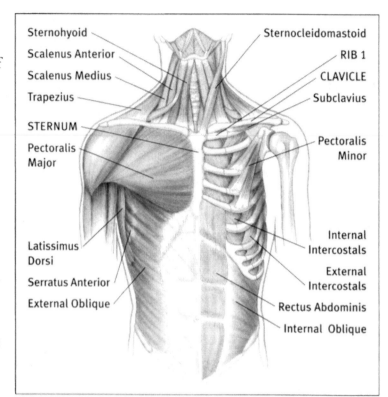

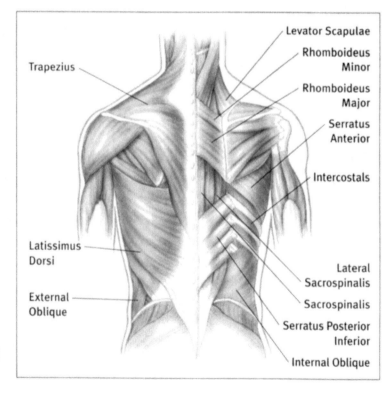

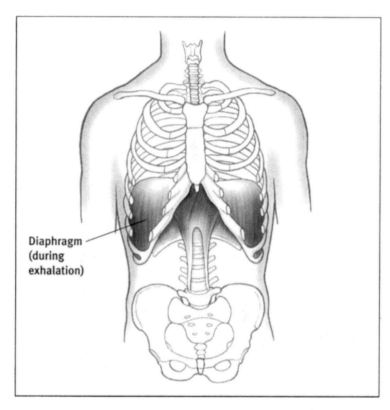

Diaphragm
(during
exhalation)

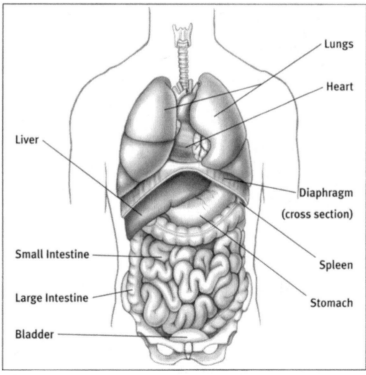

Lungs

Heart

Liver

Diaphragm
(cross section)

Small Intestine

Spleen

Large Intestine

Stomach

Bladder

any learned breathing technique. Take about 5 minutes to completely engross yourself in the experience of breathing.

As you open your eyes, begin sharing responses to the questions below. Since the intention is to reestablish a conscious link between your mind and breath, stay active in the learning process. Use the illustrations to help locate your breathing muscles.

Where in your body do you feel the breath?

Where do you notice the most movement?

Describe the rate of your breath.

Describe the length of your breath.

Describe the depth of your breath.

Describe the quality of your breath.

Describe the overall feel or texture of your breath.

Exploration II— Synchronized Breathing

One of the axioms of Partner Yoga is that all things are interdependent. Our relationship with trees and plants is a perfect example. In the

Breath

Are you looking for me? I am in the next seat.
My shoulder is against yours.
You will not find me in stupas, not in Indian shrine rooms,
nor in synagogues, nor in cathedrals:
not in masses, nor kirtans, not in legs winding around your
own neck, nor in eating nothing but vegetables.
When you really look for me, you will see me instantly—
you will find me in the tiniest house of time.
Kabir says: Student, tell me, what is God?
He is the breath inside the breath.

—Kabir

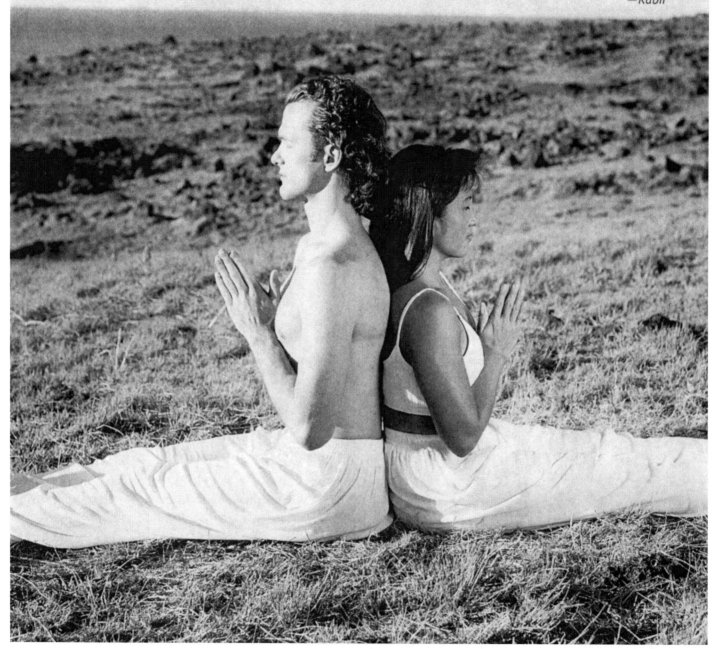

marketplace of respiration, there are two major commodities: oxygen and carbon dioxide. Fortunately, nature provides for all things. Trees and plants "inhale" carbon dioxide and "exhale" oxygen, and humans inhale oxygen and exhale carbon dioxide. It's a match truly made in heaven!

This exploration is an opportunity to consciously practice interdependence and sharing with your partner. We call it synchronized breathing.

Begin by sitting back to back with your legs straight out in front of you. Press your back gently against your partner's back, making a firm connection along the entire back side of the body. Adjust your posture until you feel that you are equally supported by and supporting your partner. Bring your palms together and rest the knuckles of the thumbs in the notch at the bottom of your breast bone. Close your eyes and begin to tune in to your own breath. Feel your ribs rise and fall against your hands. Feel your back expand and contract against your partner's.

While continuing to be aware of your own breath, begin to notice how your partner is breathing. Feel your breath against your partner's back. Take note of the rate, depth, and sound. Then slowly begin to adjust your breathing pattern to match your partner's. Invariably, one of you will have a longer breathing pattern. The point is to meet somewhere in the middle where you both feel comfortable. For the next 5 minutes (longer if you desire), allow this new shared breath to become its own creation. Stay focused and relaxed and let the breath lead the way.

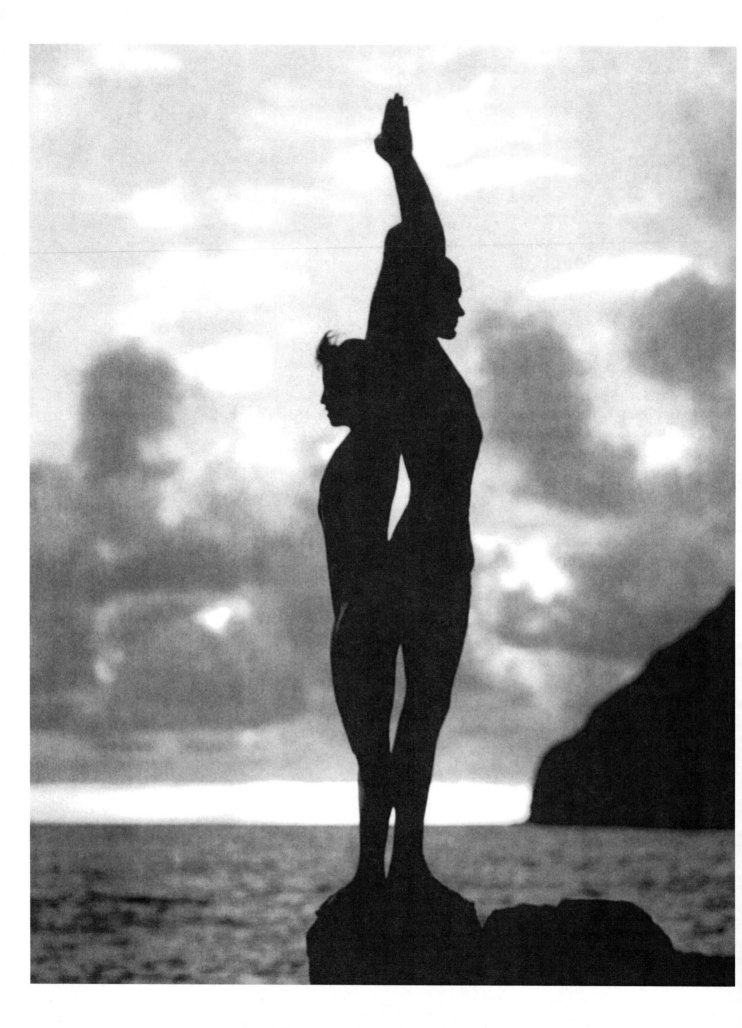

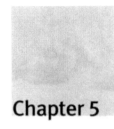

Chapter 5

Your Natural Alignment

"To know oneself as a body is more important, at this moment in history, than to read the words of all the wise men who have ever lived."

—Marco Vassi

Alignment is the dynamic process of creating harmony within yourself. When you are aligned, you are able to be more by doing less. The more aligned you are, the greater your sense of calmness and stability. Your life flows with greater ease. Alignment is about continually discovering relaxed and efficient ways of being in the world. Have you noticed how some days everything clicks, and other days you feel like you got up on the wrong side of the bed? Your alignment affects everything you do. With awareness, you can make choices in every moment that support your natural alignment.

In Partner Yoga, we ask you to explore the process of finding your own natural alignment. We are not suggesting that there is a fixed state of "perfect alignment" that everyone needs to attain. Instead, we give you general guidelines that serve as navigation tools on your journey toward natural alignment.

Before beginning a Partner Yoga session, take a moment to check in with your alignment. Face your partner, relax, and stand as you usually stand. Close your eyes and make a mental note of exactly how aligned you feel. Now open your eyes and gently observe your partner. Take turns walking around each other, or perhaps watch each other walk for a few steps. Share with each other what you have discovered about your own alignment and your partner's alignment. Stand once more in front of each other and close your eyes. Integrate what you have just learned and see if you notice a difference. Sometimes if you have been walking around or standing out of balance for a while, it feels awkward to stand aligned. This awkward feeling is a sign that your body is integrating this new information and working to make adjustments. Your brain became used to rerouting its messages because of the imbalance, and now it needs time to get used to the more aligned pathway. Always take a few moments before practicing Partner Yoga to check in with your alignment, and you will feel better as you move through the postures.

Alignment Guidelines

1. Feet: Stand with your feet parallel and about hip-width apart, weight evenly distributed. Balance your weight evenly between the heels and balls of your feet, keeping your toes relaxed.

2. Legs: Lengthen out through your legs, keeping your knees straight without locking them.

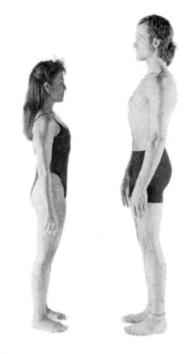

3. Pelvis: Allow your tailbone to drop toward the floor, and let your hips sit naturally over your legs.

4. Abdomen: Gently engage your lower abdominal muscles, creating a lifting feeling in the core of your body.

5. Spine: From the lift in your abdomen, feel your spine lengthening as if an invisible string is pulling you from the top of your head. Keep the central axis of your body perpendicular to the ground.

6. Chest and back: With your sternum slightly lifted, allow your chest and ribs to stay open. Widen through your back and allow your entire body to become hollow. (This creates more space for the breath to move freely.)

7. Shoulders and arms: Allow your shoulders to relax and drop away from your ears. Feel your shoulder blades gliding down your back and your arms hanging freely at your sides.

8. Head: Keep your chin parallel to the ground and relax your face and jaw.

9. Heart: Leave your pride behind and stand humbly in the present moment. Check in with your feelings, open your heart, and share with your partner.

10. Mind: Leave your judgment behind. Without attachment, become aware of your thoughts and focus your attention on the present moment.

11. Spirit: Tune in to your breath and begin to listen to your inner voice. Connect with your higher source.

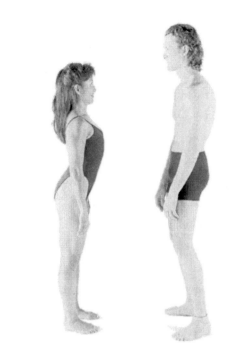

The more aware you become of your natural alignment, the more you notice when something is slightly "out." For example, something is obviously not quite right in the upper-right photo. Notice that Lori's knees are locked, her spine isn't lengthened, and her chest and back aren't open. Cain's feet aren't parallel, his knees aren't straight, and his lower abdominal muscles aren't engaged.

Since balance depends largely on alignment, achieving balance in postures becomes easier as your alignment improves. For example, keeping your foot, ankle, knee, and hip in the same line helps your balance and prevents joint strain and injury. You also want to make sure your foot presses evenly on both sides. This creates a lift in the arch and stabilizes your foot and ankle. As you move in and out of postures, maintain this foot, ankle, knee, and hip alignment.

Notice in the photo below that the

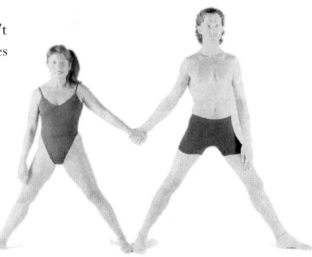

heel of one foot is aligned with the middle of the other foot. This is the proper position whenever you're stepping forward or to the side.

In knee-bending postures, like Double Warrior, your knees need to be strong and mobile. One simple knee bend involves an intricate process of bones hinging, ligaments stabilizing the movement, and menisci reducing friction. If the knee is strained, tense, or unable to hinge efficiently, there is an increased chance of injury. Other joints often come to the rescue to compensate, but this puts an increased strain on them and throws the

body's entire alignment off. To prevent knee strain, whenever you bend your knee in a standing (weight-bearing) posture, allow your knee to stay directly over your ankle and in line with your second toe. Your shin bone is perpendicular to the ground in this position. This is the most stable position for the knee. If it is difficult to keep your knee at the 90-degree angle, it is better for your knee to be slightly behind your ankle than in front of it.

An aligned body moves with greater ease and strength. You will notice as you get in touch with your natural alignment that you feel calmer and stronger. For example, lifting someone heavier than yourself requires much less strength if you take advantage of proper joint alignment and body mechanics. In a lift like the one shown below, the strength of the pose depends largely on the position of the legs

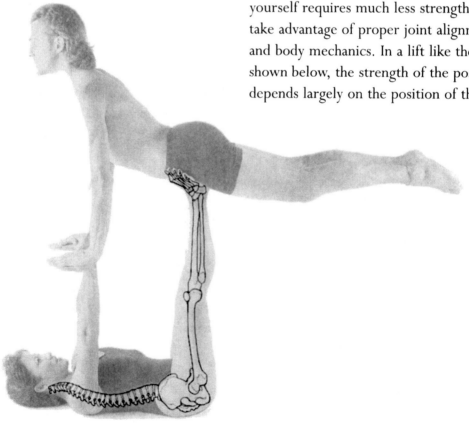

and arms. When the legs and arms are parallel to one another and perpendicular to the floor, the pose is stable and enjoyable. When the body is misaligned, the pose causes unnecessary strain and is much more difficult to execute.

A Balanced Wheel

The most obvious form of alignment is physical or structural alignment. Are you leaning your weight more on one foot? Are your shoulders hunched over? The more you connect with your partner, however, the more you will begin to see that physical alignment is only one aspect of alignment. In Partner Yoga, we look at alignment from a holistic perspective. We focus our mind (mental alignment) and stay conscious of our breath and our intuition (spiritual alignment). We address our feelings (emotional alignment) and pay attention to our physical structure and how our body works together with our partner's body (physical alignment). We have found that when we pay attention to our alignment on all of these levels, postures require much less effort and, in general, life flows with greater ease.

Visualize your whole being as a wheel with many spokes. Each spoke represents one of the integral parts of the self—the body, mind, emotions, and spirit. When all of the spokes of a wheel are properly tuned, they work together to create a strong wheel that rolls smoothly. When all of your faculties are working in harmony, like spokes of a balanced wheel, you too are strong and healthy and can roll steadily along life's sometimes bumpy road. You can accomplish more by doing less.

Of course, many of us get "bent out of shape" over the years because of socialization, stress, or challenging circumstances. For example, a dedicated athlete may overextend his physical body and pay much less attention to his mental, emotional, and spiritual alignment; a computer or business analyst may overwork her mind and dangerously neglect her body. For optimum health, it is paramount that we pay attention to all aspects of our alignment. The process of finding your natural alignment does take a little effort, however the journey is rich and the rewards are many.

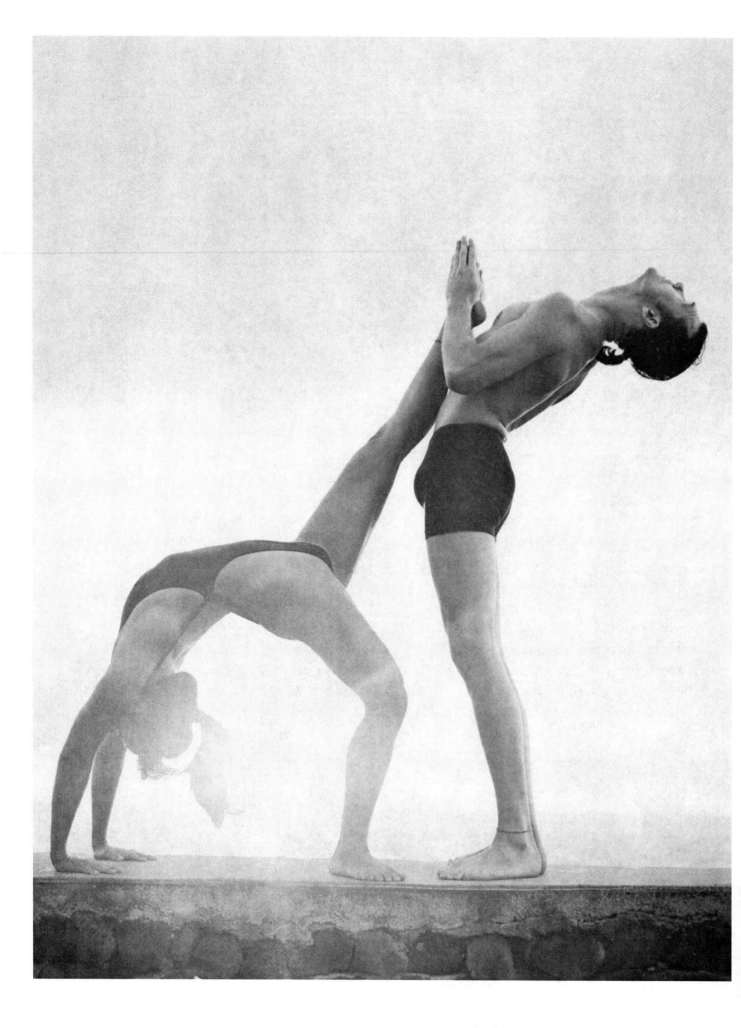

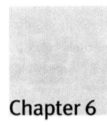

Chapter 6

Warming Up

"Yogic exercises and breathing techniques turn up your body's thermostat, purifying the physical nature with heat so that it can tolerate the extra energy produced by the emergence of the spiritual body. Energy produced in this way is often described as a bright inner fire."

—Alice Christensen, author of *Yoga of the Heart*

It's time to get moving and generate some heat. Since those first few days of gym class, most of us have been aware of the importance of warming up before physical activity. For many of us, warming up has become second nature. If you play sports, practice martial arts, or attend aerobics or dance classes, you know that instructors almost always start with some exercise that "gets the blood flowing." Actors and singers warm up their voices and face muscles to get ready for a rehearsal or performance. And writers often do warmup exercises to get in the creative flow of putting words on paper. The purpose of any warmup is to move you in the direction of your highest potential.

The practice of Partner Yoga requires that you involve your physical body as well as your mental, emotional, and spiritual "bodies." You could certainly practice the partner postures for the physical benefits alone. Yet to get the most from your Partner Yoga practice, it is necessary to involve the whole you. To move toward "whole-self" involvement, we have developed a short series of exercises that "get the blood flowing" in all of your bodies. We call it the All-Body Warmup.

Awake and Aware

We realize that the concept of an all-body warmup might be a bit of a stretch for some people. Let us clarify by explaining what it means to be "warm" in each of your bodies. Figuratively, we refer to the different bodies (physical, mental, emotional, and spiritual) as separate entities. In reality, however, there are no distinct separations between the bodies; in fact, they overlap greatly to create the unique being that is you.

At the physical level, warming up means increasing the blood supply to muscles and joints so that the physical body can perform at a higher level with less chance of injury; we call this the state of being *awake*. Being awake, however, does not necessarily mean you are warm. In order to truly be warm, your body has to be both awake and *aware*. Body awareness is a two-fold condition: First, you must be aware *of* your body (how your joints feel, where you are holding tension, and so on); second, you have to be aware *with* your body. The latter is a bit more subtle, yet no less important. To be aware with your body means that you are physically experiencing the present moment: You feel the air with your skin; you feel the floor with your feet; you sense balance, movement, and spatial relationship. In short, you are living in your body instead of merely existing in it.

In our conventional system of education, we learn about the human body intellectually, by looking at diagrams and memorizing the parts. Many people can name all the muscles in the back and shoulders, yet few can simply relax those areas of their own bodies—somatic therapists call this phenomenon sensory-motor amnesia. The ability to relax, or efficiently use, a part of the body involves controlling the appropriate muscles. This ability begins with awareness. It does not matter how strong you are; if you cannot sense a part of your own body, you will not be able to control it.

The connection between the mental body and the physical body begins with the breath. An essential part of the All-Body Warmup is strengthening the mind/body connection through awareness of your breathing.

Warming up the emotional body involves becoming conscious of what you are feeling (awake) and how your feelings manifest as outward expressions (aware). Similarly, warming up the spiritual body means being awake and aware of your breath and intuition. You are awake in your spiritual body when you are listening to your intuition, and you are aware when you can see the connection between your actions and your intuitive notions.

The All-Body Warmup

The All-Body Warmup starts with simple exercises for the feet and ankles and moves progressively up the body to the neck and head. During the 10-minute routine, all of the major joints and muscle groups are involved. As bloodflow increases to the muscles and joints, the body heats up and begins to release tension and purge toxins. This creates space for the breath to move freely. Through conscious breathing, the body and mind are then rejuvenated with fresh energy.

As you move through the exercises beginning on page 46, avoid becoming overly concerned with perfecting the physical movements. We would rather you perform the physical movements to the best of your ability and devote the remainder of your attention to the subtler aspects: breathing, noticing your thoughts, observing your feelings, and hearing your inner voice. Remember, the intention is to get warm in all of your bodies. Focus intently on feeling each movement. Notice how each movement involves and affects your entire body. Stay aware of your balance and alignment. Most important, stay relaxed and allow any tightness and tension to dissolve.

Throughout the warmup, practice letting go of the temptation to judge your performance or that of your partner. Practice accepting things as they are, including your perceived limitations and imperfections, and allow yourself to simply be present with the experience.

Invariably, you and your partner will move through the warmup at a pace that is comfortable and natural for you. Allow this pace to become a "flow" that carries you smoothly from one exercise to the next without pausing. Remember that your flow begins with your breath. If you consciously maintain a smooth and relaxed breathing pattern, your movement will also be smooth and relaxed. And if your breathing is deep, your experience and awareness will be deepened as well. Establish your natural rhythm, and allow the warmup to be a graceful dance.

Note: In the photographs beginning on page 46, we are facing different directions for the purpose of explaining the exercises from two different angles. We suggest that you and your partner warm up facing each other a few feet apart.

Honoring

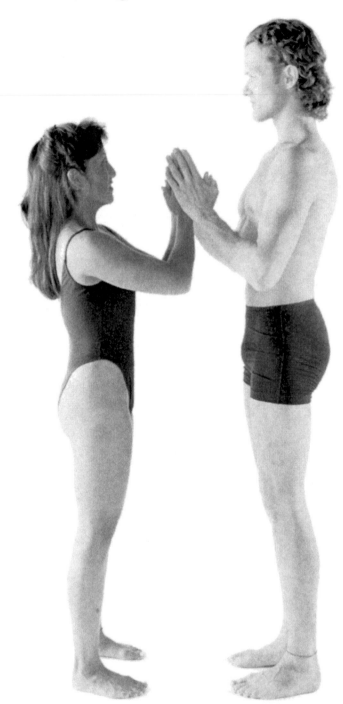

PURPOSE

- Allows you to center yourself, acknowledge your partner, and tune in to each other

TECHNIQUE

- Stand facing your partner. Bring the palm of your right hand together with your partner's right hand. Raise your left hand to the outside of your partner's right hand. We call this hand position partner namaste. Close your eyes and relax your shoulders. Notice your breathing and allow yourself to become keenly aware of the present moment. Simply be here now.

- Allow the sense of connection you feel in your hands to move slowly down your arms and into the rest of your body. Take as long as you need to feel centered and connected to your partner.

- Slowly open your eyes and look at your partner. Smile, nod, or in your own way, extend a gesture of honor and respect toward your partner.

- Slowly release your hands, take a few steps back, and get ready to move.

The Chair

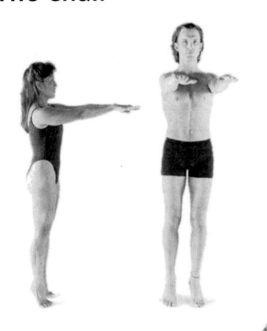

PURPOSE
* Warms up the calves and thighs
* Increases awareness of balance and body position

TECHNIQUE
* Shake out your feet and ankles and wake up your feet.

* Stand with your feet about hip-width apart. Raise your arms to shoulder height in front of you, and relax your neck and shoulders.

* Inhale, lengthen your spine, and rise up on your toes.

* Exhale and slowly bend your knees, as if sitting in a chair. Hold steady and relaxed in the chair position for three breaths.

* Come up slowly and return to the normal standing position.

* Repeat the sequence three times.

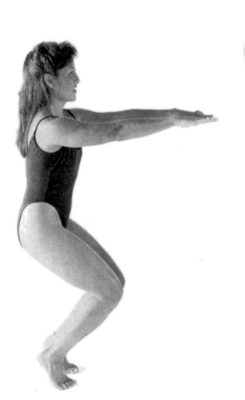

Grand Plié

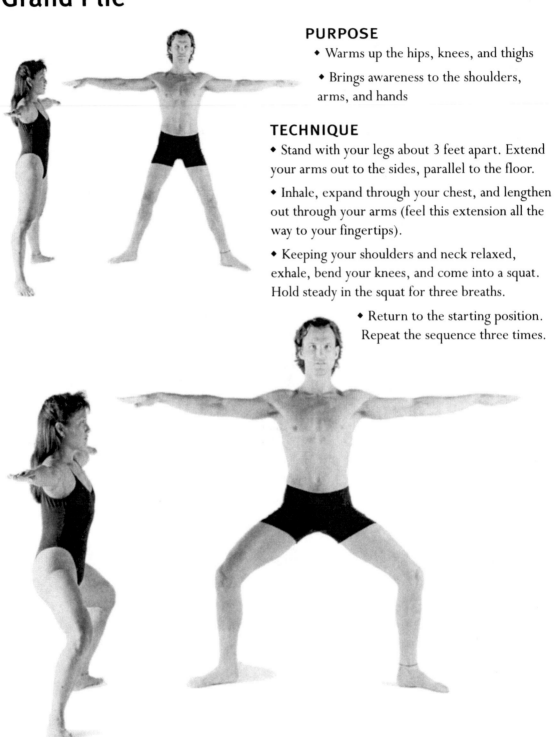

PURPOSE

- Warms up the hips, knees, and thighs

- Brings awareness to the shoulders, arms, and hands

TECHNIQUE

- Stand with your legs about 3 feet apart. Extend your arms out to the sides, parallel to the floor.

- Inhale, expand through your chest, and lengthen out through your arms (feel this extension all the way to your fingertips).

- Keeping your shoulders and neck relaxed, exhale, bend your knees, and come into a squat. Hold steady in the squat for three breaths.

- Return to the starting position. Repeat the sequence three times.

The Knee Lift

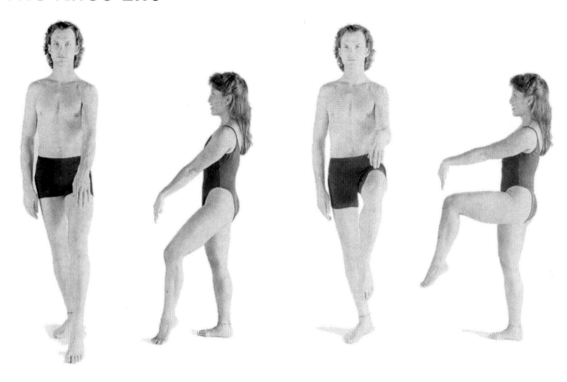

PURPOSE

* Warms up the hips and thighs

* Increases awareness of balance and grace

TECHNIQUE

* Stand with your feet about hip-width apart. Shift your weight to your right leg and step your left leg forward about 12 inches. Shake out your left arm and relax your shoulder.

* Hold your left hand over your left knee and imagine that the two are connected by a string.

* Inhale, lifting your left hand and knee simultaneously until the thigh is parallel to the floor. Exhale and slowly release back to the starting position.

* Move smoothly up and down. Repeat 10 times on each side.

Small and Large Hip Circles

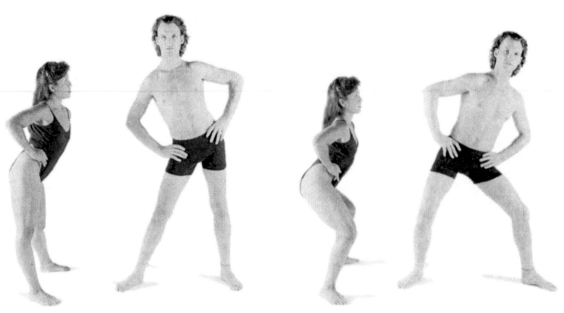

PURPOSE

- Warms up the muscles in the hips, buttocks, and lower back

- Brings awareness to the entire pelvic region

TECHNIQUE

- To do small hip circles, stand with your legs about 2½ feet apart.

- Bring your hands to your hips and begin making slow circles with your hips, keeping the movement smooth and consistent. Keep the rest of your body still and relaxed. Concentrate on feeling the movement in your hips and pelvic region.

- As you continue to circle, use your fingers to feel how the muscles of your hips and buttocks contract and relax.

- Complete 10 circles in each direction.

- To do large hip circles, step your feet out a couple of inches from position one. Allow your tailbone to sink toward the floor by bending your knees.

- Continue circling your hips, progressively increasing the size of your circles.

- Use your legs to help create more movement in your hips. Remember to keep the rest of your body relaxed. Stay focused on your hips and pelvis.

- Complete 10 circles in each direction.

Standing Cat/Cow

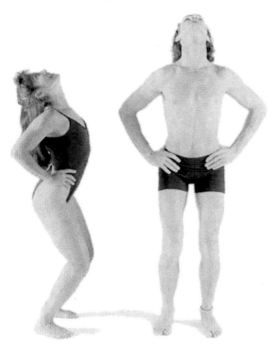

PURPOSE

• Warms up the spine and stretches the chest, shoulders, and abdominal muscles

• Increases awareness of the muscles that support the neck and spine

TECHNIQUE

• Stand with your feet about shoulder-width apart. Bend your knees slightly and bring your hands to your hips.

• Keeping length in your spine, inhale deeply as you tip your pelvis forward and arch your lower back.

• Continue inhaling as you extend the arch up your entire spine. As you arch back, keep your chest and ribs open and your shoulders relaxed.

• Feel the muscles in your back and neck contract, and feel your abdominal muscles lengthen and release.

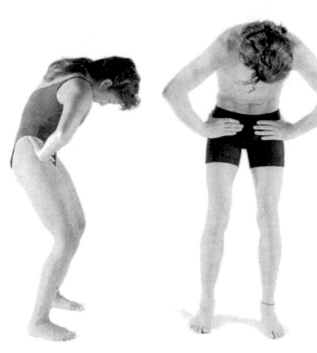

• Exhale, tuck in your tailbone, and slowly begin to bow your spine. Notice how the muscles in the front of your body contract and pull you forward, while the muscles in your back and neck stretch and release.

• Repeat 10 times.

NOTE: Always coordinate the movement with the breath—inhaling to arch backward and exhaling to bow forward.

Side Stretch

PURPOSE

- ◆ Warms up the arms and shoulders
- ◆ Stretches the ribs and intercostal muscles
- ◆ Brings awareness to the muscles along the sides of the body

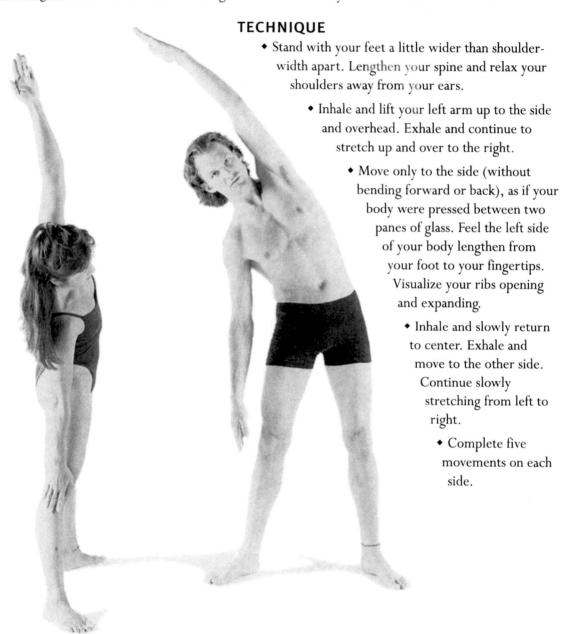

TECHNIQUE

- ◆ Stand with your feet a little wider than shoulder-width apart. Lengthen your spine and relax your shoulders away from your ears.
- ◆ Inhale and lift your left arm up to the side and overhead. Exhale and continue to stretch up and over to the right.
- ◆ Move only to the side (without bending forward or back), as if your body were pressed between two panes of glass. Feel the left side of your body lengthen from your foot to your fingertips. Visualize your ribs opening and expanding.
- ◆ Inhale and slowly return to center. Exhale and move to the other side. Continue slowly stretching from left to right.
- ◆ Complete five movements on each side.

The Archer

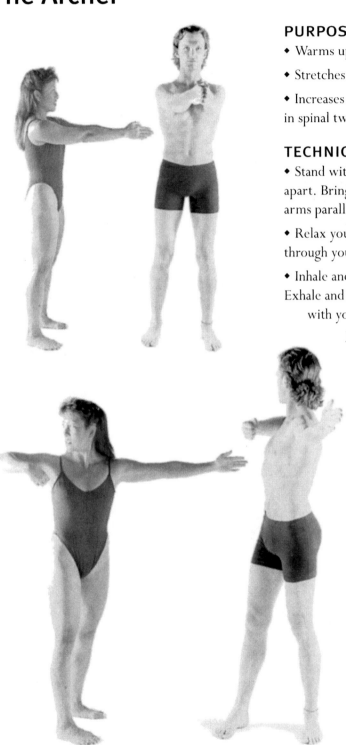

PURPOSE

◆ Warms up the upper back and shoulders

◆ Stretches the chest and ribs

◆ Increases awareness of the muscles involved in spinal twisting

TECHNIQUE

◆ Stand with your feet about shoulder-width apart. Bring your palms together, with your arms parallel to the floor.

◆ Relax your shoulders and lengthen out through your fingertips.

◆ Inhale and create length in your spine. Exhale and rotate to the right, drawing back with your right arm. Inhale and extend your right arm forward as you rotate to the left, drawing back with your left arm.

◆ Continue rotating back and forth. Imagine that you are an archer drawing back the string of a giant bow. Feel the muscles working in your shoulders and back and notice the opening in your chest and ribs. Complete 10 movements on each side.

NOTE: Always coordinate the movement with the breath—inhaling to the left and exhaling to the right.

Flicking Tension

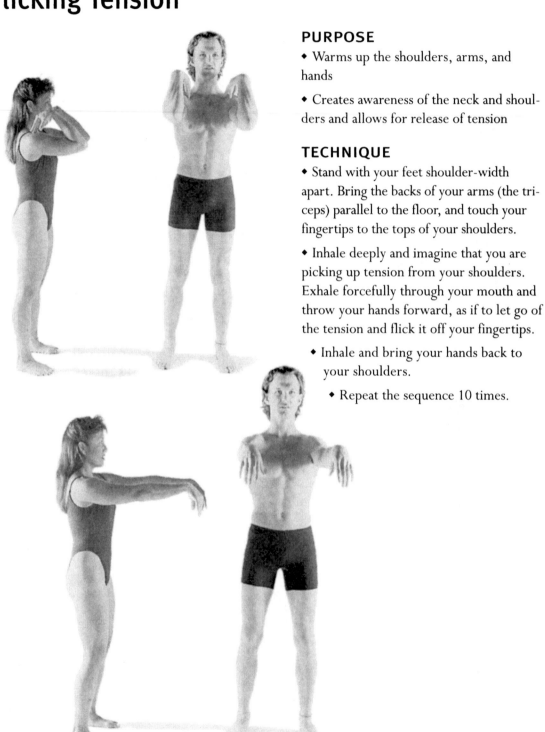

PURPOSE

• Warms up the shoulders, arms, and hands

• Creates awareness of the neck and shoulders and allows for release of tension

TECHNIQUE

• Stand with your feet shoulder-width apart. Bring the backs of your arms (the triceps) parallel to the floor, and touch your fingertips to the tops of your shoulders.

• Inhale deeply and imagine that you are picking up tension from your shoulders. Exhale forcefully through your mouth and throw your hands forward, as if to let go of the tension and flick it off your fingertips.

• Inhale and bring your hands back to your shoulders.

• Repeat the sequence 10 times.

Arms of Air

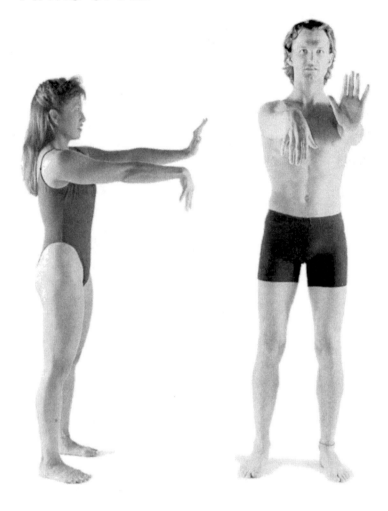

PURPOSE

♦ Warms up the shoulders, forearms, wrists, and hands

♦ Increases awareness of the body/breath connection

TECHNIQUE

♦ Stand with your feet shoulder-width apart. Raise your arms forward until they are parallel to the floor. Relax your neck and shoulders.

♦ Begin to flex and extend your wrists while keeping the rest of your body still and relaxed.

♦ Tune in to your breathing, and imagine your breath rising up your body into your arms and all the way out to your fingertips. Feel your arms becoming light as they fill with breath.

♦ Continue flexing and extending for 1 minute without lowering your arms.

Neck Stretches

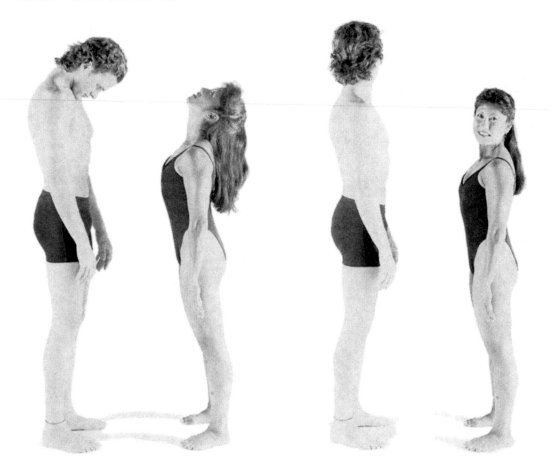

PURPOSE

◆ Warms up the neck and throat

◆ Releases tension in the shoulders and neck (primarily the trapezius muscles)

TECHNIQUE

◆ Stand with your shoulders relaxed and lengthen your neck and spine.

◆ Inhale and slowly lift your chin toward the sky. Exhale and slowly bring your chin down to your chest.

◆ Rest in this position for a moment and imagine tension melting off your shoulders and dripping down your arms and off the ends of your fingers.

◆ Continue slowly moving your head forward and back. Take note of the neck muscles as they contract and extend.

◆ Complete five stretches forward and five back.

◆ Turn your head slowly from left to right, inhaling as you come to center, exhaling as you look to the side.

◆ Keep your chin parallel to the floor and your shoulders relaxed. Feel the muscles on the sides of your neck.

◆ Complete five stretches on each side.

◆ Inhale and create length in your neck. Exhale and slowly lower your right ear toward your right shoulder. Inhale as you come back to center.

◆ Exhale and stretch down to the left.

◆ Focus on the movement of the muscles that connect the shoulders and neck.

◆ Complete five stretches on each side.

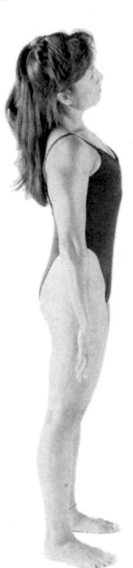
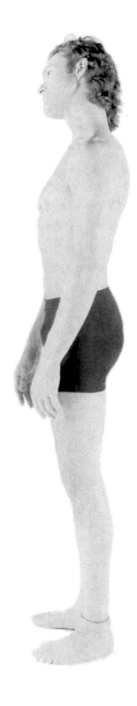

Sun Moon Union

PURPOSE

* Increases awareness of the breath/movement connection

* Facilitates equal awareness of both sides of the body

TECHNIQUE

* Stand with your legs about 2½ feet apart. Root down into your feet and lengthen up through your spine.

* Touch the tips of your thumb and forefinger together in *jnana mudra*, the seal of wisdom.

* Begin to inhale while slowly raising your arms forward. Feel as if your arms are floating upward on your breath. When your hands are just above your eyes, touch your fingertips together and hold your breath.

* Imagine that within you, you are uniting the great forces of the sun (your right hand) and the moon (your left hand).

* Exhale, turn your hands palms up, and slowly float your arms back down. Feel as if your arms are descending with the breath.

* Repeat the entire sequence three times.

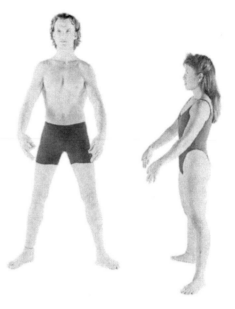

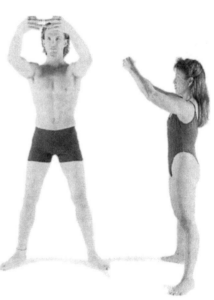

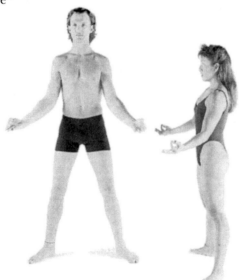

NOTE: This exercise serves as a symbol of the fundamental purpose of yoga: to create unity among opposing forces. Move slowly, and concentrate on feeling the connection between the breath and the movement.

PART TWO

PARTNER POSTURES

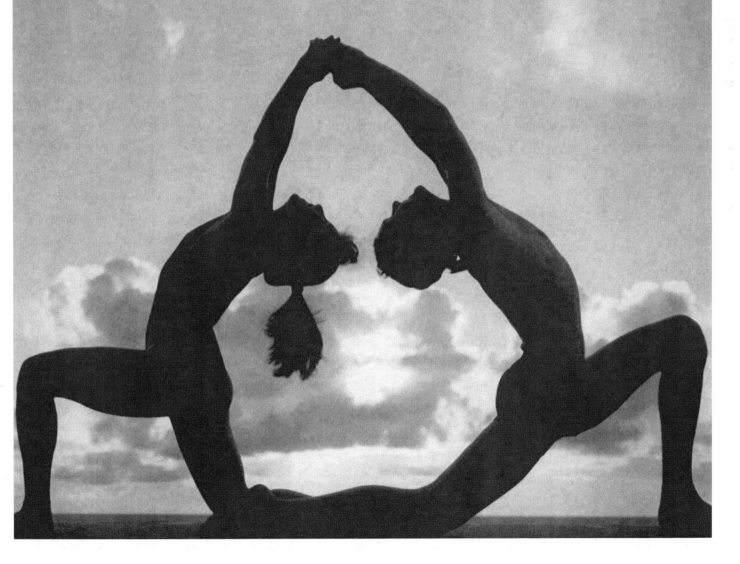

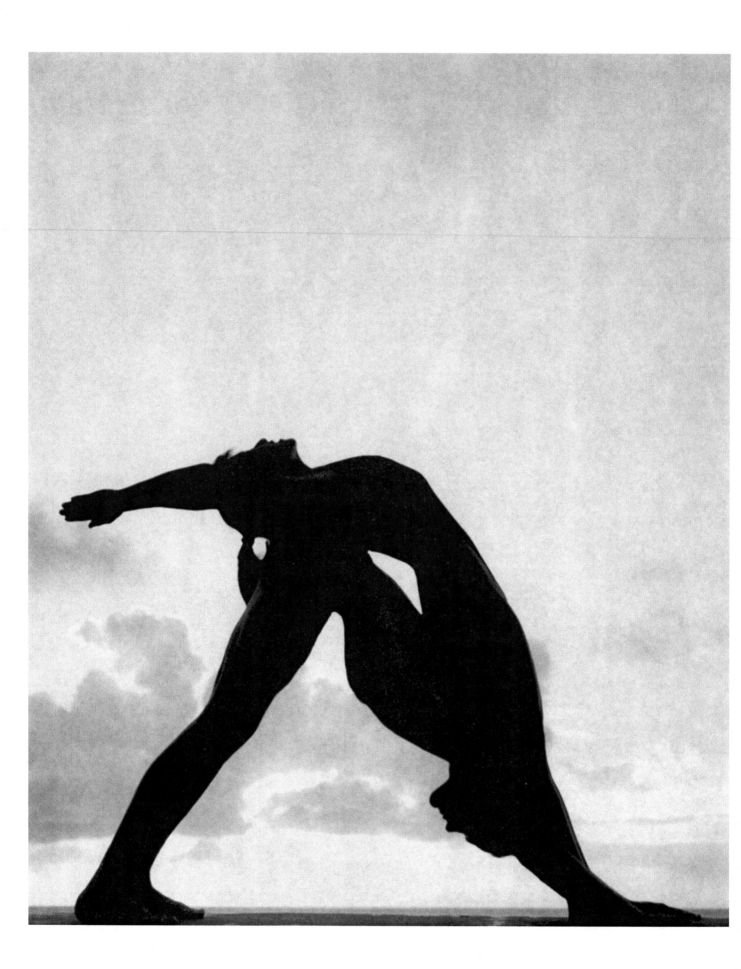

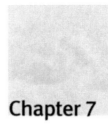

Chapter 7

Strength, Stamina, and Flexibility

"Either you reach a higher point today, or you exercise your strength in order to be able to climb higher tomorrow."

—Friedrich Nietzsche

Since the beginning of humankind, people have had to uphold a certain level of fitness just to procure the basic necessities of life. Throughout most of history, there has been little need to "exercise" to stay fit. Until recent times, if you wanted anything done, you had to exert at least a moderate physical effort to make it happen. People stayed in shape by simply going about their daily activities. Nowadays, in most industrialized countries at least, this is no longer the case. With a cell phone, a computer, and a car, you can orchestrate your entire life without so much as raising your heart rate.

In light of all our recent technological advancements, our culture is still primitive in its understanding of our basic human needs. In many ways, modern technology has made our lives easier, yet not necessarily healthier. While our living environment continues to change drastically, our bodies remain the same as they have been for thousands of years. If we are to keep up with the challenges of this changing world, we must redefine what it means to be fit.

Typically, we think of fitness only in terms of physical fitness—how fast you can run, how high you can jump, how much weight you can lift, and so on. In Partner Yoga, we address fitness from a holistic perspective that includes four different areas: physical, mental, emotional, and spiritual. We assess our overall level of fitness by taking into consideration our strength, stamina, and flexibility in each of these four areas. The optimum level of fitness will be different for each of us, depending on our personal goals and lifestyle.

To better understand the concept of holistic fitness, let's compare the fitness needs of two imaginary characters: Joe, a middle-aged office manager in Phoenix; and Elaine, a late-twenties tour guide working her first summer in the Himalayas. In Joe's busy office, he spends a good deal of his day behind a desk. By lunch, his shoulders and neck are already tense, and he suffers a mild upset stomach. By the end of the day, Joe's lower back is sore, his stomachache is worse, and he is exhausted.

On a typical day in the mountains, Elaine is responsible for leading a group of about seven tourists on a rugged 6-hour hike, often at high altitude. At the end of the day, Elaine's feet and legs are tired and tight, her shoulders and upper back are sore from the weight of her pack, and she has a mild headache.

When it comes to physical fitness, Joe's needs for strength, stamina, and flexibility are much different than Elaine's. Since Joe spends most of the day seated, he would greatly benefit from a regular practice of Partner Yoga, involving postures that invigorate the legs and hips and stretch and strengthen the neck, shoulders, and back. The practice of deep breathing would help calm his nerves and relieve the anxiety contributing to his stomachache. Elaine, on the other hand, spends all day on the move exerting herself physically. She could use a regular practice that involves relaxing partner postures that help increase flexibility in the legs, hips, chest, and back. The practice of deep breathing would increase Elaine's lung capacity, helping her absorb more oxygen at high altitudes.

Mentally, emotionally, and spiritually, Joe and Elaine's fitness challenges are surprisingly similar. Joe is responsible for overseeing the functioning of the entire office, including five employees. Elaine is responsible for providing her seven clients with a safe and fun-filled adventure. Both positions require the mental strength to make important decisions and the stamina to think clearly and stay focused for long periods. Joe needs to be mentally flexible to best manage his diverse employees and keep up with industry changes. Elaine deals with the unpredictable forces of nature and personality, and she must stay mentally flexible to account for changes in weather or whim.

In addition to meeting their physical and mental challenges, Joe and Elaine also have to be emotionally and spiritually fit. During the busy time of the year, Joe's office is under increased stress, and emotions among employees run high. To keep morale up, Joe has to muster the emotional and spiritual strength and stamina to stay positive and keep his employees inspired. To do this, he follows his intuition and comes up with creative ways of making work fun. It would be easy for Joe to lose his temper and simply treat his employees like workers. Instead, he finds the strength and flexibility to act compassionately and treat his employees like real people.

Leading tourists into the high mountains can be risky business. To avoid unnecessary dangers, Elaine uses her intuition for guidance even more than she uses her compass. Listening constantly to her spiritual voice requires extreme diligence and spiritual stamina. Elaine's position also requires her to be emotionally strong in the face of danger, yet sensitive and caring toward clients who may be scared or suffering from altitude sickness. And since she deals with people of diverse ethnic and religious backgrounds, Elaine has learned to be tolerant and spiritually flexible.

After reading these examples, think about how the concept of holistic fitness fits into your own lifestyle. Look closely at your personal needs for strength, stamina, and flexibility in each of the four areas (physical, mental, emotional, and spiritual). As you practice the partner postures, make a note of the postures that best serve your specific needs and the needs of your partner.

Home Base

As you practice the partner poses, take time to rest when you need it. Depending on the pose you are in and how you are feeling at the time, you can take a break by moving into any one of the three resting poses, beginning on page 64. Think of these poses as home, and come back to them anytime you like.

The section on standing poses follows the three resting poses. In each of the standing partner poses, we offer a suggested duration of time for holding the pose. These time durations are only suggestions, and we ask that, when in doubt, you do what feels true for you. For simplicity, in all of the photos we refer to Cain as Partner One and Lori as Partner Two. This organization continues throughout the book.

Resting Poses

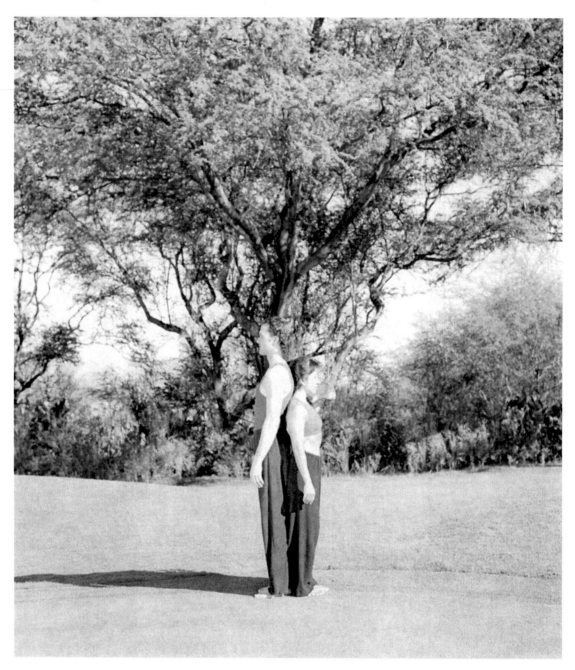

Mellow Mountain Pose
Simply stand back to back with your feet about hip-width apart. Breathe and relax.

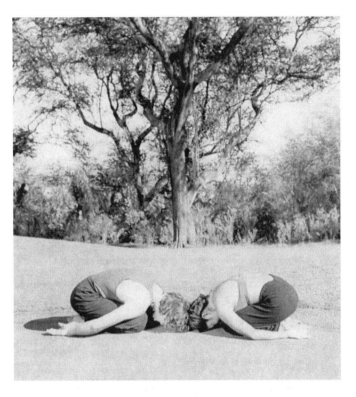

Child Pose

Kneel in front of your partner with your forehead on the ground and the top of your head touching your partner's head. Relax your shoulders and neck. Breathe. This is a wonderful counter-pose to do after intense back bends.

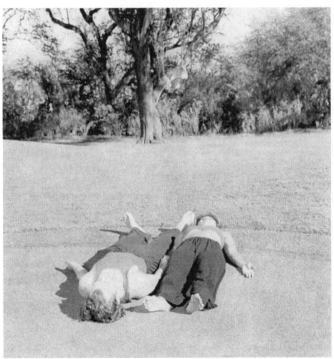

Corpse Pose

The Corpse Pose is one of our favorites. Lie side by side, facing opposite directions. Lengthen your spine and align your entire body. Let your feet drop out to the sides, and relax your hands palms up. Breathe and let go.

Twin Peaks

Twin Peaks is formed as two partners come standing back to back in *Tadasana*, the Mountain Pose. This basic pose is the foundation for all standing Partner Yoga postures.

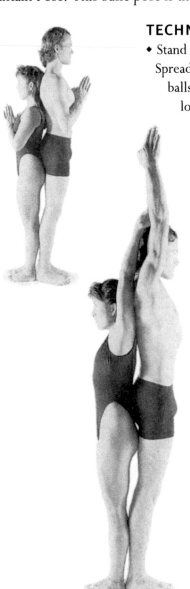

TECHNIQUE

- Stand back to back with your feet parallel, about hip-width apart. Spread your toes and distribute your weight between the heels and balls of your feet. Lengthen out through your legs without locking your knees. Allow your tailbone to drop and feel how your hips align over your knees.

- Visualize a golden cord attached to the top of your head and gently pulling your entire spine toward the sky.

- Relax your shoulders, and bring your palms together in front of your heart.

- Inhale and extend your arms overhead with your palms together.

- Keeping your arms straight, link hands (or link one partner's hands to the other's arms, depending on the height difference) and open through your chest and shoulders.

- Breathe smooth and deep and hold the pose for 15 to 30 seconds.

Partner Pointers

Evenly distribute your weight on both feet.

Reach up through your fingertips and allow gravity to pull your shoulders down away from your ears.

Share your insights on body alignment with your partner.

Benefits

Centers the mind ◆ Increases awareness of posture ◆ Exposes structural imbalances in the body

Double Moon

Double Moon is an adaptation of the classic yoga pose *Chandrasana*. This crescent-shaped pose provides a wonderful side stretch and opens the ribs for deeper breathing.

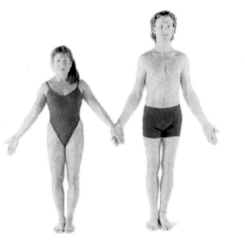

TECHNIQUE

◆ Stand side by side, about 3 feet from your partner. Connect your inside hands and lengthen out through the spine.

◆ Inhale and raise the outside arms up and overhead and begin to extend up and in toward your partner.

◆ Allow your hips to move slightly away from each other as your hands connect overhead. Make sure your spine stays long and avoid collapsing the ribs on the inside.

◆ Breathe and hold the pose for 15 to 45 seconds. Repeat on the opposite side.

Partner Pointers

As you bend to the side, keep your entire body moving on the same plane. Imagine that you are pressed between two pieces of rice paper; if you lean forward or back, the paper will tear.

As you reach toward your partner's hands, initiate the movement from your spine and allow your shoulders to stay relaxed.

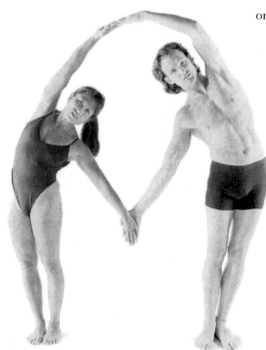

Benefits

Opens the sides of the body ◆ Creates space in the rib cage, making deep breathing easier ◆ Increases awareness of hip and spinal alignment

The Table

This forward-bending pose is great for opening the shoulders and chest and releasing tightness in the backs of the legs. The Table is simple enough that it can be done anywhere. We often relax using this pose at airports between long flights.

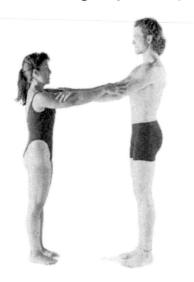

TECHNIQUE

• Stand facing your partner about 2 feet apart.

• Link arms just above the elbow and begin slowly bending forward while taking small steps away from each other.

• Bring the tops of your heads together and slide your hands out to your partner's shoulders.

• Lengthen your spine and flatten your back by extending your buttocks away from the top of your head.

• Exhale and relax your shoulders and allow your chest and ribs to open toward the floor.

• Allow your breathing to be smooth and deep. Hold the pose for 30 to 60 seconds.

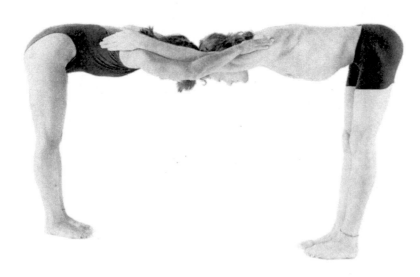

Partner Pointers

The Table works best when your back is parallel to the floor and your legs are perpendicular to the floor.

Allow chest expansion without constricting the space between your shoulder blades.

Benefits

Stretches backs of legs and buttocks ◆ Strengthens the muscles in the lower and mid-back ◆ Opens the chest and shoulders

Double Chair

The Double Chair is a powerful counterbalance pose that builds trust and nurtures teamwork. The Double Chair is great for developing leg strength and proper spinal alignment.

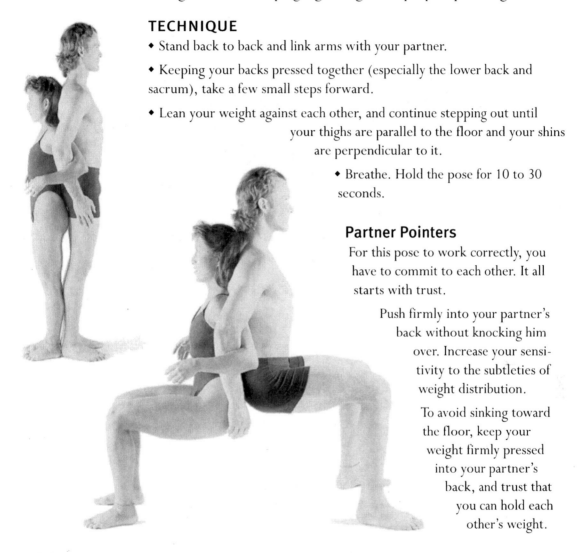

TECHNIQUE

♦ Stand back to back and link arms with your partner.

♦ Keeping your backs pressed together (especially the lower back and sacrum), take a few small steps forward.

♦ Lean your weight against each other, and continue stepping out until your thighs are parallel to the floor and your shins are perpendicular to it.

♦ Breathe. Hold the pose for 10 to 30 seconds.

Partner Pointers

For this pose to work correctly, you have to commit to each other. It all starts with trust.

Push firmly into your partner's back without knocking him over. Increase your sensitivity to the subtleties of weight distribution.

To avoid sinking toward the floor, keep your weight firmly pressed into your partner's back, and trust that you can hold each other's weight.

CAUTION: To avoid excessive strain on your knees, make sure the front of your shinbone is perpendicular (90 degrees) to the floor.

Benefits

Develops trust and teamwork ♦ Strengthens the thigh muscles ♦ Corrects slouching by lengthening the spine ♦ Increases concentration and awareness of balance

Double Downward Dog

The Double Downward Dog is a playful adaptation of the traditional Downward Facing Dog pose, *Adho Mukha Svanasana*. This invigorating pose develops arm and shoulder strength and helps both partners maintain correct alignment and proper form.

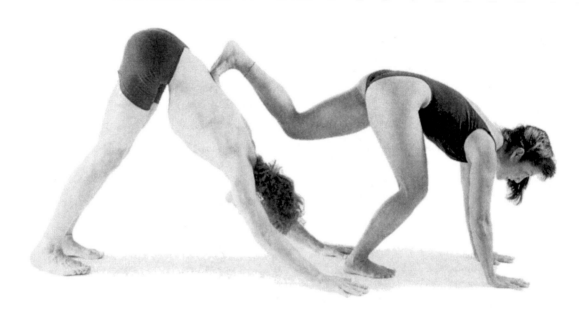

TECHNIQUE

• Partner One, position yourself on your hands and knees with your toes flexed and the balls of your feet on the floor. Keep your feet parallel, about hip-width apart, and your hands shoulder-width apart.

• Spread your fingers wide and push your palms into the floor. Straighten your legs and arms and lift into an upside-down V position. Lengthen through your spine and neck.

• Gently flex your thigh muscles and push your heels toward the floor.

• Partner Two, stand between One's hands. Bend your knees, place your hands on the floor in front of you about shoulder-width apart, and step one foot up to the center of One's lower back.

• Balance your weight and then step up to One's back with your other foot. Straighten your arms and legs and maintain length in your spine.

• Both partners, breathe into your chest and back. Hold the pose for 15 to 30 seconds. Come down slowly and rest in Child Pose.

• Switch positions and repeat the pose.

Partner Pointers

Make sure your arms and torso are about parallel to your partner's.

Partner One, maintain a strong upside-down "V" position by keeping your thigh muscles engaged and lower back lengthened.

Partner One, allow Two's weight to transfer into your legs. This will naturally give your nice stretch and take some weight off your arms.

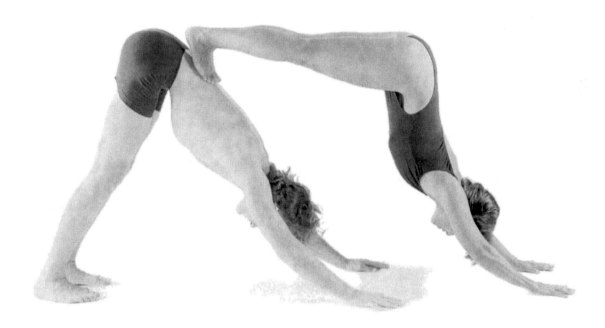

NOTE: Depending on differences in height or flexibility, Partner Two may need to adjust her hand position forward or back. The placement of her feet, however, remains the same.

CAUTION: Double Downward Dog is not recommended for people with high blood pressure or a history of stroke.

Benefits

Strengthens the shoulders, upper back, and thighs ◆ Stretches the calves, hamstrings, and buttocks ◆ Opens the chest and increases lung capacity ◆ Increases bloodflow to the brain and helps to clarify the mind ◆ Develops endurance and willpower

Downward Dog Back Bend

This invigorating pose uses the Downward Facing Dog as a platform for safely practicing the back bend. The Downward Dog Back Bend creates a beautiful form that opens the chest and fills the lungs with *prana*, the vital life force or breath.

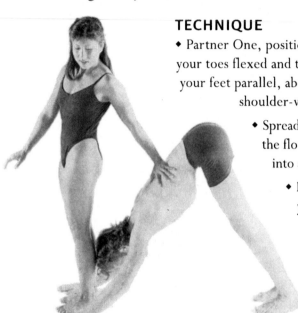

TECHNIQUE

+ Partner One, position yourself on your hands and knees with your toes flexed and the balls of your feet on the floor. Keep your feet parallel, about hip-width apart, and your hands shoulder-width apart.

+ Spread your fingers wide and push your palms into the floor. Straighten your legs and arms and lift into an upside-down V position.

+ Lengthen your spine and neck. Gently flex your thigh muscles and push your heels toward the floor.

+ Partner Two, stand with your feet together between One's arms. Reach back with one hand and support yourself as you slowly lean the backs of your thighs and your buttocks onto One's upper back.

+ Partner Two, inhale and create length in your spine. Tuck your tailbone and push your hips slightly forward. Exhale and slowly arch backward so that your upper back contacts One's lower back and sacrum.

+ Surrender into the pose by relaxing your head back and stretching your arms overhead. (This actually takes weight off of One's hands and transfers it to his legs, which makes the pose easier and helps bring his heels down.)

+ Hold the pose for 15 to 30 seconds. Come out slowly and rest in Child Pose. Switch positions and repeat.

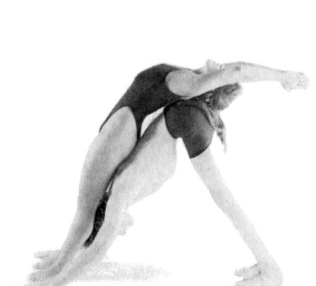

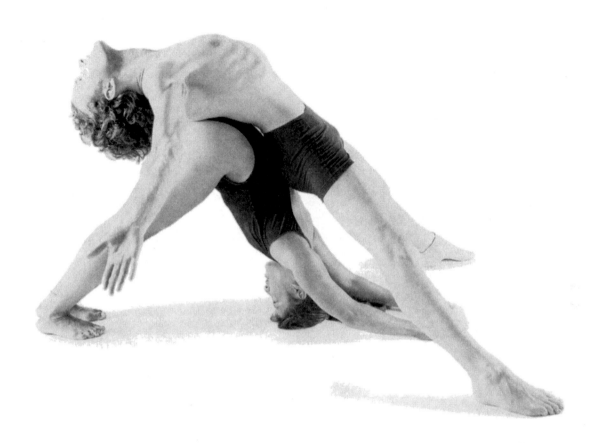

VARIATION: If one partner is considerably taller than the other (as in our case), a variation may be needed when performing the back bend. When the taller partner goes into the back bend, he spreads his feet as wide as it takes for his mid-/upper back to rest against his partner's sacrum and lower back. This maintains the structure of the pose by transferring his body weight into his partner's legs instead of her arms.

CAUTIONS: Downward Dog Back Bend is not recommended for those with high blood pressure or a history of stroke. Back bending is not recommended for those with acute spinal or neck injuries.

Benefits

Partner One
Strengthens the shoulders, upper back, and thighs ◆ Stretches the calves, hamstrings, and buttocks ◆ Balances the endocrine system ◆ Develops power and stamina

Partner Two
Stretches the entire spine ◆ Opens the belly, chest, shoulders, and neck ◆ Stimulates the heart and lungs ◆ Deepens trust and connection between partners

The Pump

The Pump is a counterbalance pose that stretches and strengthens the entire back side of the body. This pose is an adaptation of the traditional standing forward bend, *Padahastasana*, which literally means "hand to foot pose."

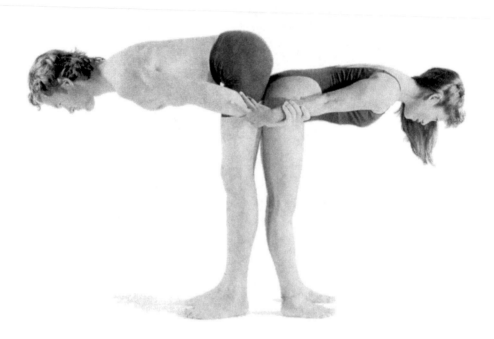

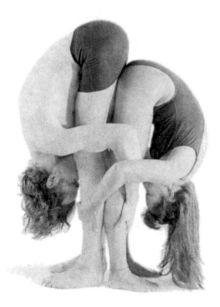

TECHNIQUE

• Stand back to back in Twin Peaks (see page 66). Link hands and relax your arms and shoulders.

• Inhale and lengthen out through the spine. Exhale and slowly begin to bend forward. (At this point, you may need to take a small step forward to keep your balance.)

• Press your buttocks firmly together by pulling in on your hands. Continue to bend forward, maintaining a long spine and flat back.

• As you move farther into the forward bend, allow your hands to rotate so that you hold each other's wrists (adjust your hand position up or down on the arms as needed).

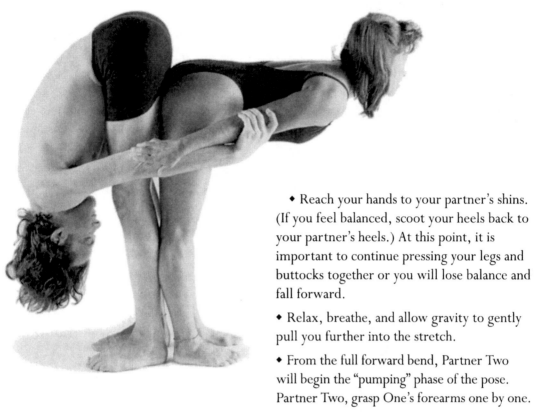

◆ Reach your hands to your partner's shins. (If you feel balanced, scoot your heels back to your partner's heels.) At this point, it is important to continue pressing your legs and buttocks together or you will lose balance and fall forward.

◆ Relax, breathe, and allow gravity to gently pull you further into the stretch.

◆ From the full forward bend, Partner Two will begin the "pumping" phase of the pose. Partner Two, grasp One's forearms one by one.

◆ Maintaining a flat back, inhale and slowly begin to lift your body parallel to the floor. Keep your arms active and your buttocks pressed together.

◆ Look straight ahead and hold your body there for a couple of breaths. Lower down slowly.

◆ Partner One, repeat the sequence.

◆ Since The Pump has various stages, allow 30 seconds to 2 minutes to complete the whole sequence.

Partner Pointers

Always move slowly and with control, especially when your spine is involved.

It is common to fall forward with this pose when you're first learning the balance. If you begin to fall, make sure you let go of your partner's hands and catch yourself. It may take a few attempts.

Benefits

Strengthens calves, buttocks, and lower-back muscles ◆ Stretches the entire back side of the body (primarily the hamstrings) ◆ Develops balance and awareness of body position ◆ Increases blood-flow to the brain

Standing Straddle

The Standing Straddle is a variation of The Pump. This wide stance opens the hips and stretches the insides of the legs as well as the hamstrings and buttocks.

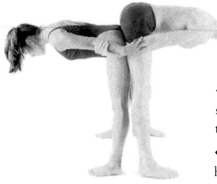

TECHNIQUE

• Stand back to back with your feet about 3 feet apart. Link hands and relax your arms and shoulders.

• Inhale and lengthen out through the spine. Exhale and slowly begin to bend forward. (At this point, you may need to take a small step forward to keep your balance.)

• Press your buttocks firmly together by pulling in on your hands. Continue to bend forward, maintaining a long spine and flat back.

• As you move farther into the forward bend, allow your hands to rotate so that you hold each other's wrists (adjust your hand position up or down on the arms as needed).

• Reach your hands to your partner's. At this point, it is important to continue pressing your legs and buttocks together, or you will lose balance and fall forward. You can also reach to your partner's shins or thighs (without pulling back on your partner's knees).

• Relax, breathe, and allow gravity to gently pull you farther into the stretch. Hold the pose for 30 to 60 seconds.

Partner Pointers

Always move slowly and with control, especially when your spine is involved.

It is common to fall forward with this pose when you're first learning the balance. If you begin to fall, make sure you let go of your partner's hands and catch yourself. It may take a few attempts.

Benefits

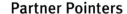

Strengthens calves, buttocks, and lower-back muscles ◆ Stretches the entire back side of the body (primarily the hamstrings) ◆ Develops balance and awareness of body position ◆ Increases blood-flow to the brain

Double Warrior B

Traditionally called *Virabhadrasana*, this pose gets its name from a famous tale in Hindu mythology. It is said that Lord Shiva pulled a strand from his matted hair and created *Virabhadra*, the courageous warrior who would lead his army against evil.

TECHNIQUE

♦ Stand back to back in Twin Peaks (see page 66).

♦ Step your feet out to the side, about 3½ feet apart. Turn one foot to the side, and keep the other foot facing forward so that your feet form a right angle.

♦ Link hands with your partner and raise your arms to shoulder height. Pull gently toward your partner to create a connection between your backs. Lengthen out through your fingertips and open your chest.

♦ Exhale and bend your front knee so that your thigh is parallel to the ground, and your shinbone is perpendicular. You may need to step back with your back leg to achieve the proper alignment. Keep your chin parallel to the floor and look out over your front hand.

♦ Breathe. Hold the pose for 10 to 30 seconds.

♦ Switch sides and repeat.

Partner Pointers

Imagine that your entire body is growing longer, especially your spine, legs, and arms. Keep your shoulders relaxed and imagine cords attached to your fingers that pull outward to stretch your arms and open your chest.

Do not lean forward or backward. Keep your spine perpendicular to the floor.

Stay aware of your feet. Instead of merely standing on your feet, think of standing *with* your feet.

Benefits

Strengthens muscles in the legs and shoulders ♦ Stretches the hips and inner thighs ♦ Produces feelings of grounding and centering ♦ Opens the chest and back

The Umbrella

The Umbrella is a powerful forward bending pose that strengthens the quadriceps while stretching the hamstrings, calves, and buttocks.

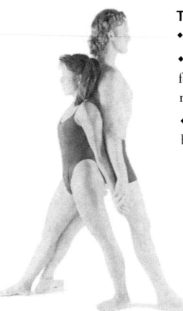

TECHNIQUE

◆ Stand back to back in Twin Peaks.

◆ Step your right foot forward and your left foot back until your feet are about 3 feet apart. Connect hands with your partner, and maintain contact with your partner's back and buttocks.

◆ Inhale and lengthen out through your spine. Exhale and start to bend forward at the hips.

◆ As you move down, rotate your hands and hold your partner's wrist or forearm (slide your hands up or down on the arms as needed). Keep your arms taut, and pull the back of your legs and buttocks together. Extend your chest out over your knee and relax your shoulders and neck.

◆ Breathe. Hold the pose for 20 to 50 seconds. Come out of the pose slowly and with control.

◆ Repeat on the other side.

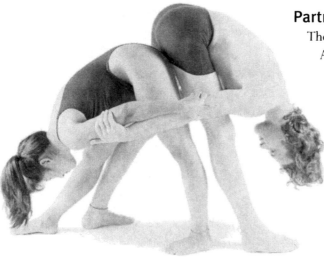

Partner Pointers

The balance in this pose can be tricky. Adjust your foot position as needed to create the most stability.

Remember, partner postures only happen when you work together. Find balance and strength by helping your partner do the same.

Benefits

Strengthens muscles in the legs and buttocks ◆ Stretches the hips and inner thighs ◆ Produces feelings of grounding and centering ◆ Opens the chest and back

Double Seated Forward Bend

The Forward Bend, *Pascimottanasana*—*pascima* means "back" and *uttana* means "extension"—lengthens the spine and stretches the entire back side of the body. This posture also massages the internal organs, increasing abdominal circulation and improving digestive health.

TECHNIQUE

◆ Sit facing your partner with the soles of your feet touching.

◆ Inhale and lengthen your spine and neck. Exhale and begin bending slowly toward your partner from your hips.

◆ Reach to your partner's hands, wrists, or forearms (use a belt or strap if needed).

◆ Maintain length in your spine as you breathe and relax forward into the pose. Focus on allowing your belly to move toward your thighs, and your chest toward your knees, rather than forcing your head to go down first.

◆ Hold for 30 to 60 seconds. Release hands, bend your knees, and come up slowly.

Partner Pointers

Always use the breath to help you move deeper into the pose. As you inhale, allow your torso to rise and lengthen, and as you exhale, simply relax and let gravity take over.

Think of the arms as an extension of the spine. Let the reaching of your hands originate at your tailbone.

NOTE: If you have tight hamstrings, as many people do, you might try bending your knees slightly (using a belt or strap). This will take some of the pressure off the back of your legs and still provide a good stretch.

Benefits

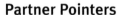

Stretches and invigorates the whole back side of the body ◆ Promotes spinal health and alignment ◆ Stimulates the abdominal organs

Butterfly Forward Bend

The Butterfly Forward Bend is a simple pose that works wonders for opening the hips and stretching the insides of the thighs. Yogis believe that this pose releases fear stored in the pelvic region.

TECHNIQUE

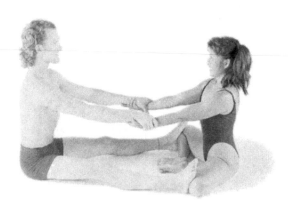

• Partner One, sit facing your partner with your legs slightly bent. Partner Two, sit close to One's feet and bring the soles of your feet together.

• Slide your feet in close to your body and allow your knees to relax toward the floor.

• One, straighten your legs and place your feet on Two's knees. Both partners, connect hands and relax your shoulders and neck.

• Two, inhale, push your sitz bones (ischial tuberosities) into the floor, and lengthen out through your spine. Exhale and begin to bend forward from your hips as you fold your arms into your body.

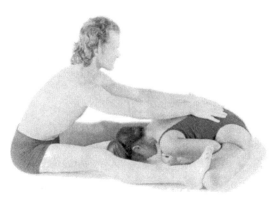

• One, as Two's head clears your arms, extend forward and rest your hands on her lower back.

• Both partners, allow yourselves to sink into the pose as far as you feel comfortable and relaxed. Breathe. Hold the pose for 30 seconds to 2 minutes.

• Switch positions and repeat the pose.

Partner Pointers

Partner One, if Two's knees are far from the floor, put your feet on top of her thighs and let the weight of your legs push gently down. Find the foot position that works best for you and your partner.

Partner Two, as you bend forward, you can keep your arms folded into your body (as in photo above) or extend them forward toward One's hips. Do what feels best for you.

Benefits

Partner One

   Stretches the hip rotators and hamstrings ◆ Releases tension in the lower back and shoulders ◆ Lengthens the spinal column

Partner Two

   Opens the hips and inner-thigh muscles ◆ Massages the abdominal organs and relieves gas/constipation ◆ Releases fear and emotional tension

Double Butterfly

The Double Butterfly is a relaxing pose that opens the hips and aligns the spine.

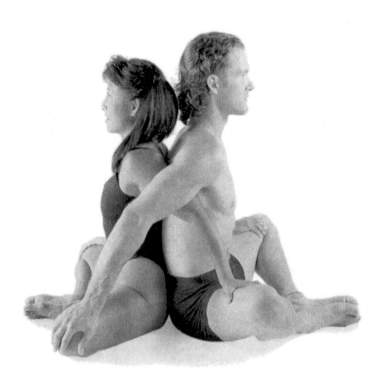

TECHNIQUE

◆ Sit back to back. Bring the soles of your feet together about 6 inches in front of you.

◆ Inhale and reach your hands back to your partner's knees. Exhale and gently press your partner's knees toward the floor.

◆ Relax your hips, thighs, and ankles. Breathe. Hold the pose for 30 seconds to 2 minutes.

Partner Pointers

Keep your back pressed firmly against your partner's back.

Relax your chest and shoulders.

Adjust the location of your feet until you feel comfortable and relaxed.

Benefits

Opens the hips and inner thighs ◆ Helps prepare you for Lotus Pose and other cross-legged positions ◆ Releases fear and locked emotions

The Diamond

The Diamond is a powerful pose for opening the hips, hamstrings, and rib cage. This lustrous pose is formed when two partners face each other in the traditional *Janu Sirasana*, literally "head to knee pose."

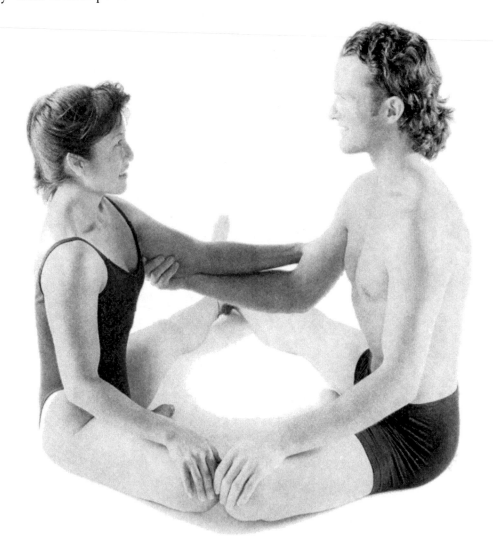

TECHNIQUE

• Partner One, sit facing your partner with your right leg stretched out to the side, and bring the sole of your left foot to your right inner thigh.

• Partner Two, face your partner and mirror this position, touching knee to knee and foot to foot.

• Both of you, hold your partner's elbow on the side of the outstretched leg.

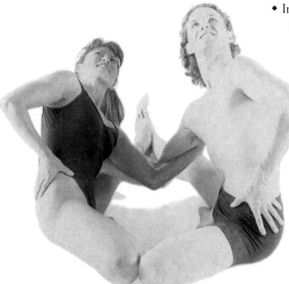

• Inhale and place your free hand on your hip and lengthen your spine. Exhale and begin to bend toward your outstretched leg.

• Lift your free arm up and over your head, then reach toward your toes. Pull in gently on your partner's elbow, and turn your chest and head toward the sky.

• Breathe and relax. Hold the pose for 30 to 60 seconds. Come out of the pose slowly and repeat on the other side.

Partner Pointers

There is a tendency to collapse the ribs when bending to the side. This is easily avoided by maintaining length in the spine. Think of increasing the distance between your floating ribs and the top of your hip.

As you look toward the sky, there is a tendency to tense up. Remember to stay relaxed in your shoulders and neck.

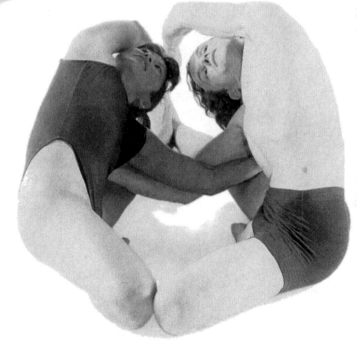

Benefits

Opens the hips, hamstrings, and inner thighs ◆ Expands the rib cage and intercostal muscles ◆ Creates space in the chest and allows more room for the lungs to expand

Butterfly Fish

The Butterfly Fish blends a hip-opening forward bend with a heart-opening back bend.

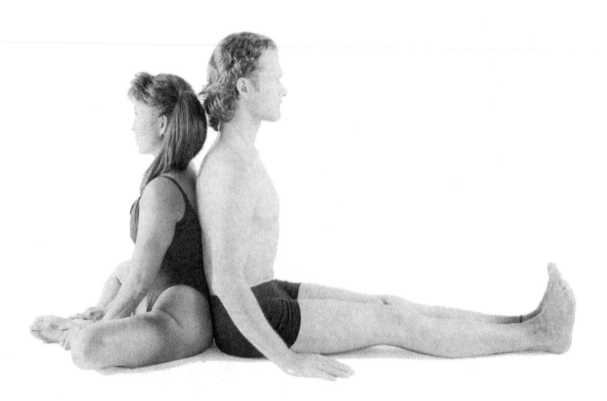

TECHNIQUE

♦ Sit with your backs firmly pressed together. Partner One, extend your legs straight out in front of you. Partner Two, bring the soles of your feet together in Butterfly.

♦ Both partners, inhale and lengthen your spine.

♦ Partner Two, exhale and slowly bend forward from the hips while walking your hands out in front of you.

♦ Partner One, maintain contact with Two's back as you move slowly into your back bend.

♦ Bring your palms together and extend your arms overhead. Breathe together and relax.

♦ Hold the pose for 30 to 60 seconds. Come up slowly and switch positions.

Partner Pointers

Partner One, be sure to keep length in your neck as you drop your head back. This will prevent kinks or strain.

Partner One, you can decrease the intensity of your back bend by sliding a few inches away from your partner. You can also place your palms together over your heart. This will lessen the stretch placed on the upper back.

Partner Two, you can move your feet toward or away from your body to find the most beneficial stretch. Do what feels best for you. Also, don't be concerned with whether or not your head touches the ground. The bend happens in the hips. Always focus on moving your belly and chest forward and then down. Your head will follow later.

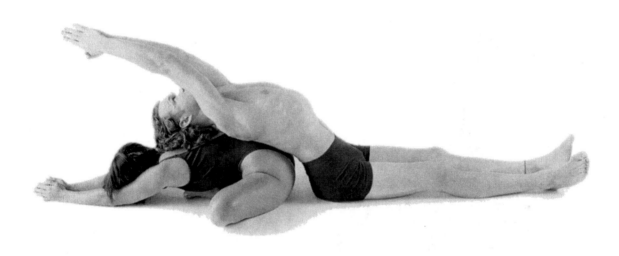

Benefits

Partner One

Opens the chest, throat, shoulders, and ribs ◆ Tones and invigorates the spine ◆ Releases stagnant energy from the heart area

Partner Two

Stretches the inner thighs and deep hip muscles (external rotators) ◆ Lengthens the spine and releases tension in the lower back ◆ Releases tension and fear stored in the pelvis

Starfish

A sister pose of the Butterfly Fish, the Starfish is a powerful pose inspired by the natural splendor of the Hawaiian coastline. While one partner stretches forward in a straddle, the other opens back in *Matsyasana*, the traditional Fish Pose.

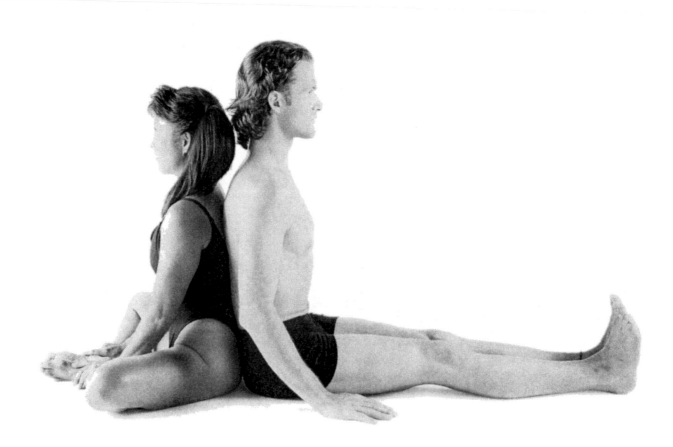

TECHNIQUE

◆ Sit with your backs firmly pressed together.

◆ Partner One, extend your legs straight out in front of you. Partner Two, sit with the soles of your feet touching.

◆ Partner Two, slide your legs out to a straddle position. Both partners, inhale and lengthen your spine.

◆ Partner Two, exhale and slowly bend forward from the hips while walking your hands out in front of you. Let your chest and belly move toward the floor as you feel comfortable.

◆ Partner One, maintain contact with Two's back as you move slowly into your back bend. Open your arms to the side and reach your hands to Two's feet.

◆ Breathe together and relax. Hold the pose for 30 to 60 seconds. Come up slowly and switch positions.

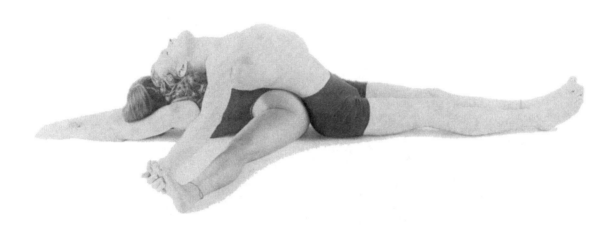

Partner Pointers

Keep in mind that the finished Starfish posture requires a certain degree of flexibility. The point is not to get overly concerned with doing the physical posture perfectly. Instead, concentrate on moving deeper into the posture mentally, emotionally, and spiritually—you'll find that the flexibility will follow.

NOTE: Partner One, to avoid pushing Two into her forward bend too quickly, you can support yourself with your hands on the floor to lower yourself slowly into the back bend.

Benefits

Partner One
   Relieves tension in the neck ◆ Opens the chest, heart, and shoulders ◆ Gives a sense of expansion and calmness

Partner Two
   Stretches muscles on the insides of the legs ◆ Invokes a sense of surrender and release

Forward Bend Fish

The Forward Bend Fish is a combination of two traditional poses, *Pascimottanasana* and *Matsyasana*; hence the pose's nickname, "Paschi Matsy."

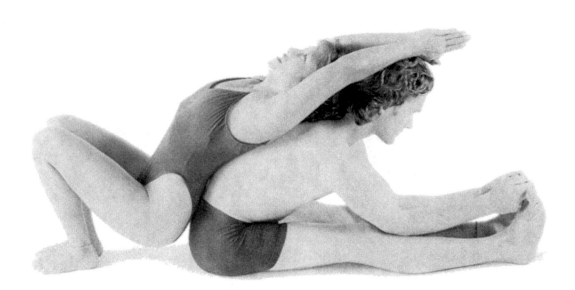

TECHNIQUE

◆ Partner One, sit with your legs extended out in front of you. Inhale and lengthen your spine and neck. Exhale and begin bending forward from the hips. Reach toward your feet and grasp your big toes. Maintain length in your spine as you exhale and relax forward into the bend.

◆ Partner Two, sit back to back with One in a squatting position. Adjust your position up or down so that your head rests on One's upper back. Inhale and extend your arms overhead with the palms together. Exhale, extend your legs, and allow yourself to relax into a gentle back bend.

◆ Hold the pose for 30 to 60 seconds. Come out of the pose slowly and switch positions.

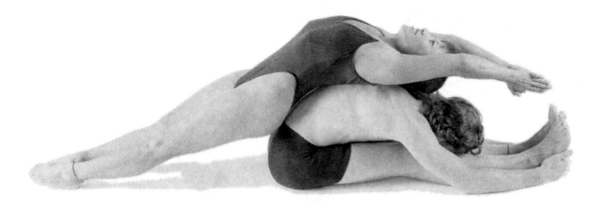

Partner Pointers

Partner One, if you cannot reach your toes, use a belt or strap until your flexibility increases (old ties work well, too).

Partner Two, if you feel uncomfortable extending your legs in the back bend, you can remain in a squatting position and still benefit from the pose.

ADVANCED VARIATION: Partner Two, for an extra challenge, you can practice Paschi Matsy with your legs in lotus position.

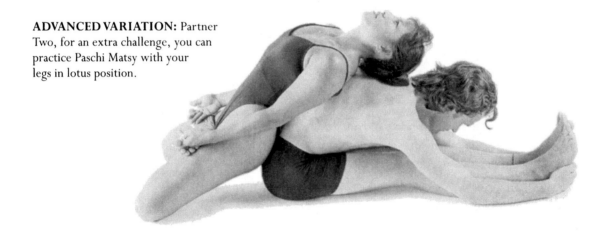

Benefits

Partner One
   Stretches and invigorates the back side of the body ◆ Promotes spinal health and alignment ◆ Stimulates the abdominal organs

Partner Two
   Releases tension in the shoulders and neck ◆ Expands the ribs and promotes deep breathing ◆ Tones and invigorates the spine

Massage Table I

The Massage Table is an all-time Partner Yoga favorite. In this dynamic pose, both partners enjoy a relaxing massage, free of charge!

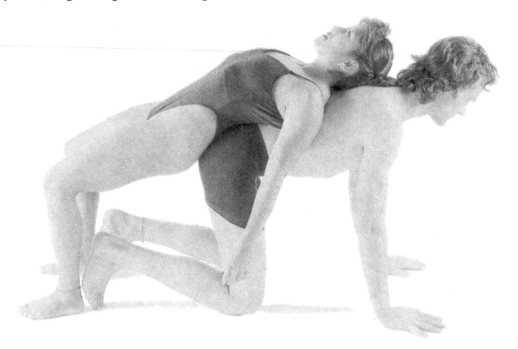

TECHNIQUE

◆ Partner One, begin on your hands and knees. Place your hands under your shoulders and spread your fingers wide. Lengthen your spine and flatten your back. Think of yourself as a strong base for your partner to lie on, like a massage table.

◆ Partner Two, gently recline onto One's back. Relax your neck and let your head rest in the middle of One's upper back. Relax your arms to the sides. Close your eyes, breathe, and enjoy the massage.

◆ Partner One, inhale, slowly arch your back, and look up. Think of stretching the entire front side of your upper body.

◆ Exhale and begin bowing your back by pushing your mid-back toward the sky. Tuck your tailbone and bring your chin to your chest.

◆ Partner Two, extend your arms over your head and lengthen through your spine.

◆ Partner One, continue this arching and bowing as you breathe long and deep; always arch as you inhale and bow as you exhale. Allow your breathing to dictate the movement.

◆ Continue the pose for 1 to 2 minutes. Come out of the pose slowly and switch positions.

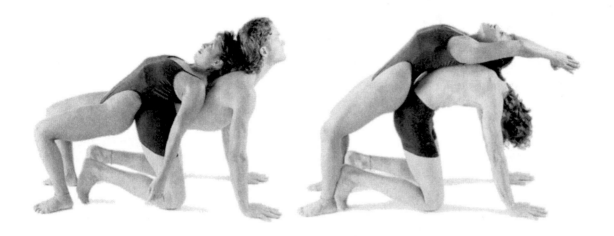

Partner Pointers

Partner One, place a towel or blanket under your knees for padding. As you arch and bow, close your eyes and visualize each vertebra moving. This will increase awareness of the spine and improve range of motion.

Partner Two, focus on maintaining long, deep breathing through the pose. This will help relieve tension and naturally open your chest and ribs.

Partner Two, you may need to slide higher or lower on One's back to find the perfect location. Some people even find that to avoid bumping their partner's head, they need to slide their head slightly to the side as the base partner arches back. As always, experiment to find what works best for you and your partner.

NOTE: You can leave your arms at your sides (see photo at left), or bring them overhead with your palms together (see photo at right). Do what feels right for you.

Benefits

Partner One
    Tones the arms and abdominal muscles ◆ Increases range of motion in the spine ◆ Strengthens the lower and mid-back

Partner Two
    Releases tension in shoulders and neck ◆ Opens the chest and heart region ◆ Invokes a feeling of softness and surrender

Massage Table II

The Massage Table II is a variation that allows the top partner to experience a deeper back bend in a safe and supported manner.

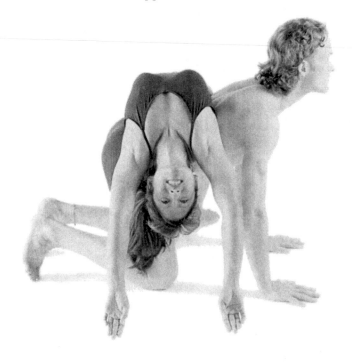

TECHNIQUE

◆ Partner One, perform the same movements as in Massage Table I.

◆ Partner Two, begin in the same position as Massage Table I. Keeping contact with One's back, slowly walk to the side until you are perpendicular to One. Adjust your position so that you rest on One's mid-back. Extend your hands overhead and allow your head to drop back gently.

◆ Breathe, relax, and enjoy the ride.

◆ Partner One, once Two is in position, you may begin slowly arching and bowing as you did in Massage Table I. Again, initiate the movement from your breath; inhale as you arch and exhale as you bow. Continue the pose for 30 to 60 seconds. Come out of the pose slowly and switch positions.

Partner Pointers

Partner Two, if extending your arms overhead puts too much strain on your back, place your palms together over your heart. This takes some of the weight off the spine while still maintaining a nice stretch.

Benefits

Partner One
Tones the arms and abdominal muscles ◆ Increases range of motion in the spine ◆ Strengthens the lower and mid-back

Partner Two
Safely opens the front side of the body while protecting the spine and neck ◆ Stretches the arms and shoulders and releases tension ◆ Develops trust between partners

Double Hurdler

The Double Hurdler is a twisting bend that lengthens the sides of the body from the hips to the fingertips.

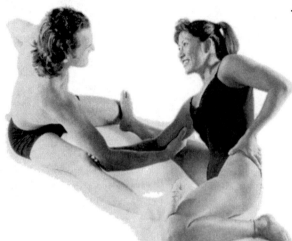

TECHNIQUE

◆ Sit face to face, about one leg length apart. Straighten your right leg toward your partner and bend your left leg out to the side.

◆ Slide toward each other until your right foot touches the top of your partner's left thigh. Adjust your position so that together your legs form a rectangle. Reach to your partner's right elbow with your right hand.

◆ Inhale and reach your left arm up and over your head. Exhale and reach toward your right foot with your left hand. Gently turn your head and chest toward the sky.

◆ Breathe. Hold the pose for 20 to 60 seconds. Release slowly and switch sides.

Partner Pointers

To create a fuller twist, gently increase the pull on your partner's arm.

As you move deeper into the pose, keep your rib cage open and your breathing smooth and deep.

CAUTION: If you've had knee problems, or if you feel strain or pain in your knees, use special caution when doing this posture.

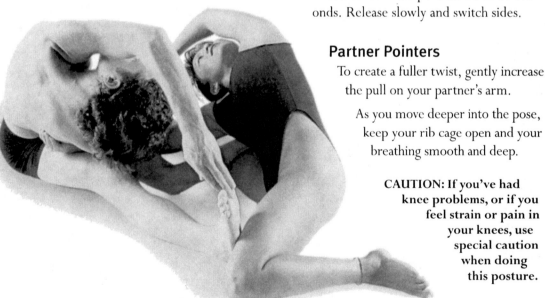

Benefits

Stretches shoulders and upper-back muscles ◆ Opens hips and hamstrings ◆ Expands the chest and opens ribs

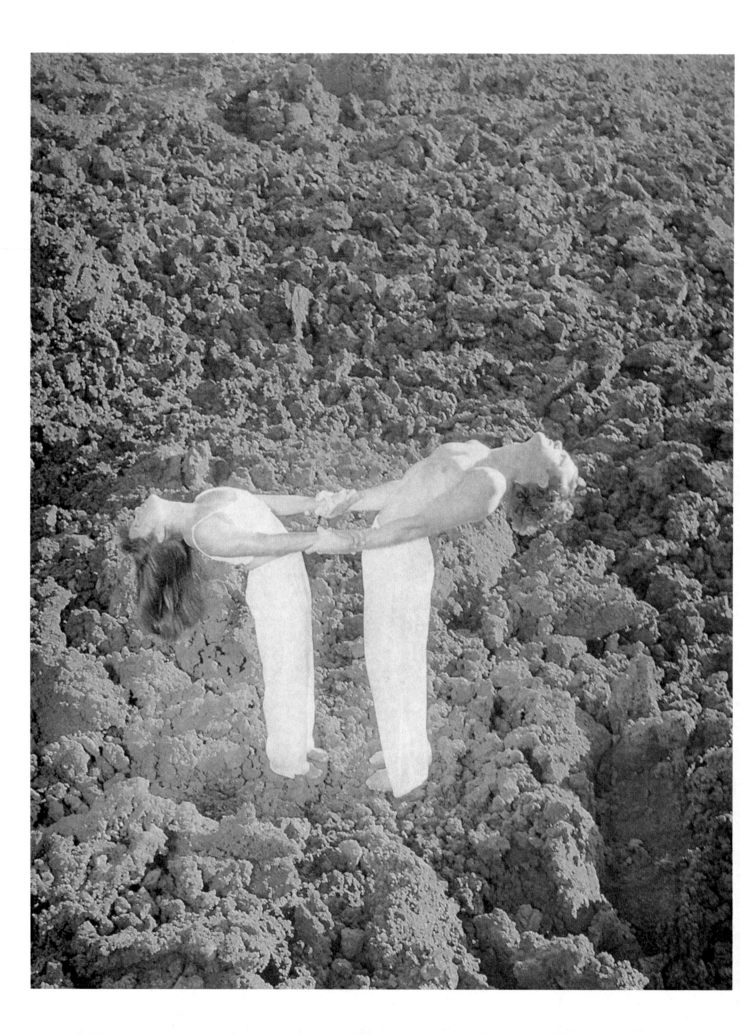

Chapter 8

Surrendering in Trust

"Gaze into the fire, into the clouds, and as soon as the inner voices begin to speak, surrender to them, don't ask first whether it is permitted or would please your teachers or father, or some god. You will ruin yourself if you do that."

—Hermann Hesse, author of *Demian*

In chapter 7, you practiced some of the basic Partner Yoga poses for developing strength, stamina, and flexibility. While practicing these poses, you may have noticed that certain positions or circumstances brought up stronger feelings than others. Perhaps you felt fear or anxiety, or even doubted your (or your partner's) ability to complete a difficult movement. These kinds of feelings are common in Partner Yoga. Often, students find it challenging to trust their partners to hold their weight or support them in a counterbalance posture. Other times, students find it challenging to allow themselves to let go emotionally and share an intimate moment with their partners. Of course, there are always a few students who just go for it, without fear or hesitation. The fact is that practicing Partner Yoga requires a certain degree of trust and surrender. In this chapter, we invite you to explore trust and surrender as you practice the following poses.

On page xvi, we list the Axioms of Partner Yoga. The first axiom reads, "All things are interdependent." Six more axioms follow, yet this first axiom is the central truth around which the entire practice of Partner Yoga is built. Every pose, every principle, and every exercise was created with this axiom in mind. You might say that Partner Yoga is a model for better understanding our lives and the world around us, and in our lives and the world around us, all things are interdependent.

Ironically, we live in a culture that supports independence as a sign of strength and freedom. We learn that it is better to "do it yourself" rather than surrender control and rely on anyone else. In our striving to be strong and independent, we sometimes forget how inherently interdependent we are on a multitude of circumstances, resources, and people. Partner Yoga is about learning to surrender your need to control, and learning to trust that you are part of a larger interdependent network that supports all life.

For example, let's say you want to build your own home. First, you are dependent on good soil and weather conditions to produce quality trees. Next, you rely on the lumber mill to cut straight boards, the metal factory to make good nails, and the hardware store to sell hammers and levels. At this stage of the project, imagine the huge web of people and resources already involved in building only the frame of your "do it yourself" home. Clearly, this is no independent project. Without even knowing it, you have trusted hundreds of people and surrendered more control than you realize. By no means is this a sign of weakness; it simply shows that you indeed are part of a larger system.

Partner Yoga reconnects you with the beauty of interdependence in your life. All of the postures are mutually supportive. As you move through your practice, you experience the power of interdependence. The more you surrender and trust, the stronger you feel and the more peaceful and relaxed you can be. Learning to trust and surrender is not about giving up your power—it's about connecting to the most powerful source of all. When you trust Life and let go of the need to be in total control, you start feeling connected, understood, and supported. This feeling is the foundation for living your truth and finding fulfillment.

As you practice the poses in this chapter, keep an open dialogue with your partner. In The Fountain pose, for example (see page 98), each partner depends on the other for support in a counterbalance posture. If you don't combine your efforts, both of you will topple. Knowing that your partner is half-responsible for supporting the pose may bring up issues of trust and surrender. If one or both of you are fighting to stay in control of your own independent balance, you will struggle. Someone always seems to be pulling a little too much or not enough, as if you are working against each other. (This is a common theme in many relationships as well.) Instead, trust and surrender is about giving in to each other and creating a balanced posture together. You are directly experiencing what it means to be interdependent. As you move into the following poses, work together. Stay open and patient. And most important, have fun in the process.

Weeping Willow

This gentle side bend releases tension in the neck and shoulders, and builds the confidence necessary for practicing more advanced forward- and back-bending counterbalance postures.

TECHNIQUE

◆ Stand side by side about 3 feet apart. Link inner hands and lengthen up through the spine.

◆ Take a small step toward your partner as you inhale and lean your upper body away from him.

◆ Exhale as you bend fully to the side. Adjust the position of your hands as needed.

◆ Continue to lengthen your spine as you bend away from your partner. Hold for 30 to 60 seconds, then gently release and switch to the other side.

Partner Pointers

Keep your ribs as open as possible on the leaning side. This is achieved by continually lengthening the spine and both sides of the body as you bend to the other side.

Relax your neck, and allow your head to move as a natural extension of your spine.

Benefits

Increases lateral flexibility of the spine ◆ Strengthens and opens intercostal muscles ◆ Fosters trust and prepares partners for other counterbalance postures

The Fountain

Like drinking fresh spring water, back bending is a great way to rejuvenate the body. The Fountain pose irrigates the spine, opens the heart, clarifies the mind, and allows your life energy to flow.

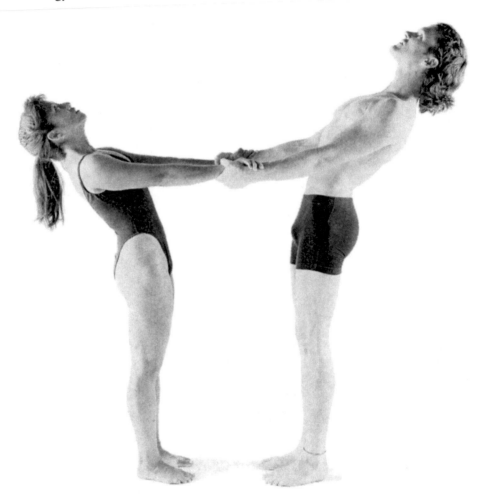

TECHNIQUE

• Stand facing your partner about a foot apart. Bring your hands to your partner's wrists in a firm, yet relaxed hold.

• Inhale as you begin to gently lengthen your spine and lean back.

• Lift from your sternum and allow your tailbone to drop.

• Press your hips toward each other, and deepen your back bend as you exhale.

• Breathe deeply and relax into the pose. Hold for 10 to 20 seconds and come up slowly.

Partner Pointers

Always be careful with your neck. Maintain length in your neck, avoid straining, and stay relaxed.

Allow your shoulders and arms to relax. Avoid bending your elbows and using arm strength to hold yourself up.

The more you relax and use your partner's counterweight to find your own balance, the deeper you will be able to stretch.

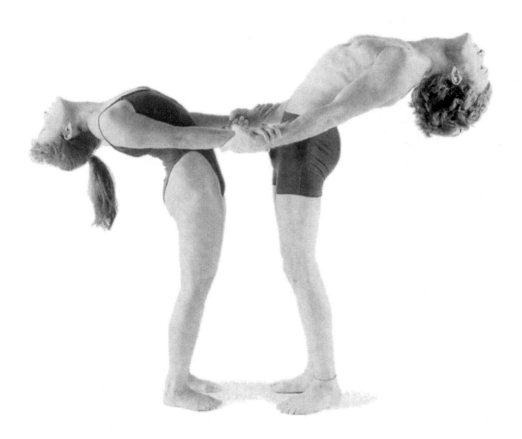

CAUTIONS: Always warm up thoroughly before practicing a back bend. Move in and out of back bends gradually, and never force yourself beyond your ability. If you have heart trouble, high blood pressure, spinal injuries, or other serious illnesses, or if you are pregnant, consult a health professional before practicing back bends.

Benefits

Builds energy and courage, enhances mood, and lifts spirit ◆ Opens the chest and abdomen and facilitates deep breathing ◆ Increases flexibility of the spine ◆ Opens intercostal muscles ◆ Improves balance and concentration

The Gateway

This pose combines the traditional Warrior pose, *Virabhadrasana*, with an expansive side bend. The Gateway invigorates your body and enlivens your courageous spirit.

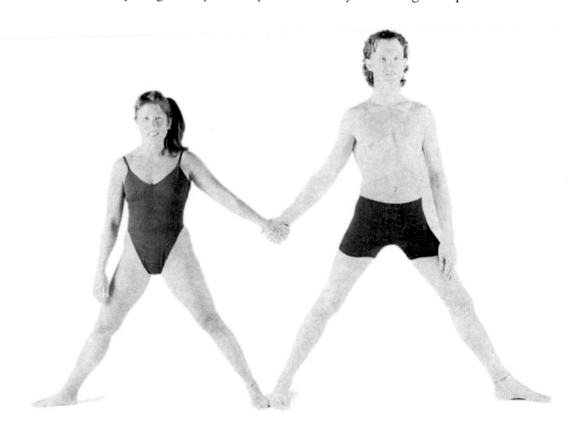

TECHNIQUE

• Begin by standing side by side, with the outer edges of your feet touching and hands linked. With your outer foot, step out to the side about 4 feet, pointing your foot in the direction you just stepped. The foot touching your partner's foot remains facing forward.

• Bend the knee of your outer leg until your shinbone is perpendicular to the ground. Adjust the distance between your feet if necessary to create that 90-degree angle.

• Inhale and begin bending in toward your partner while reaching your free hand overhead to touch your partner's hand. Exhale, relax your neck, and look toward the sky. Hold this pose for 10 to 20 seconds, breathing normally.

• Release slowly, and spend a few breaths in your beginning position before moving to the other side.

Partner Pointers

Make sure both heels are placed firmly on the ground and that your knee stays directly over your ankle or slightly behind it.

Keep your tailbone tucked and avoid leaning forward or back.

Relax your shoulders, lifting from your spine and sternum rather than your arms.

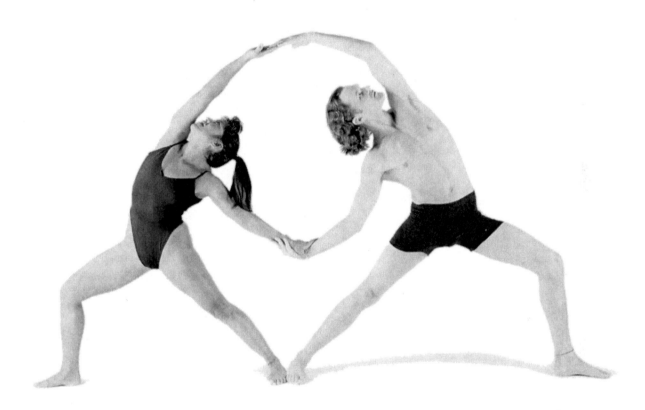

Benefits

Increases lateral flexibility of the spine ◆ Stretches and opens intercostal and abdominal muscles ◆ Tonifies abdominal and pelvic organs ◆ Stretches the inner thighs and strengthens the legs

The Backpack

This is one of our favorite traveling poses. It is a great pose to practice after sitting anywhere for an extended period of time. The Backpack combines a standing forward bend, traditionally called *Uttanasana*, with a relaxing back bend.

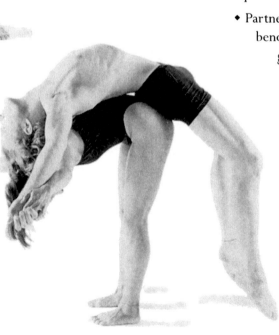

TECHNIQUE

◆ Stand back to back with your partner. Lengthen your spine, link arms, and breathe normally.

◆ Partner Two, get ready to lift Partner One over your back. This lifting process is more about leverage than strength. If you find the right placement of your buttocks on your partner's back, you will be able to lift with greater ease. Partner One, align your buttocks with Two's lower back.

◆ Partner Two, inhale deeply and slowly bend forward as you exhale, lifting Partner One onto your back.

◆ Stay in this position for a few breaths to gain your balance and find the best back-to-back contact before moving on. Sometimes Partner One will have to slide up or down Partner Two's back to find a relaxed and balanced position.

◆ Partner Two, exhale deeply and bend all the way down to the ground, lifting your tailbone to the sky and lengthening your spine. Stretch the top of your head toward the ground.

◆ Slowly release your partner's hands and let your partner rest freely on your back and sacrum. Place your hands on the ground. Hold the pose for 15 to 45 seconds.

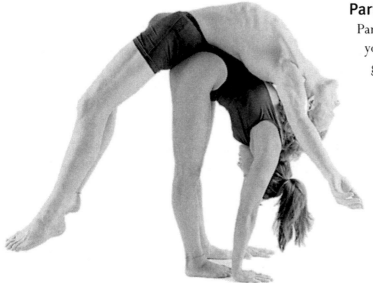

Partner Pointers

Partner Two, pay attention to your feet and keep them evenly grounded. Keep your toes relaxed and active. Remember that your feet are the solid base upon which the entire pose builds.

Partner Two, support One's hips with your hands to prevent him from falling as you begin to stand up.

VARIATION: If you feel like an extra challenge, practice the bow variation over your partner's back. Set up the same way you would have for the regular backpack pose.

When you are lying on your partner's back in a relaxed and balanced position, reach back with your hands and hold your own ankles. Once again, you may have to adjust your position on your partner's back for optimum balance.

Press the insides of your knees toward each other, relax your spine, and breathe deeply.

Partner One, you can place your hands behind your legs to pull your body toward your legs and release your spine farther.

This variation opens your chest farther and gives your legs an extra stretch.

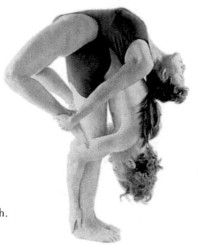

CAUTIONS: Always warm up thoroughly before practicing a back bend. Move in and out of back bends gradually, and do not force beyond your ability. If you have heart trouble, high blood pressure, spinal injuries, or other serious illnesses, or if you are pregnant, consult a health professional before practicing back bends.

Benefits

Partner One

Opens the chest and abdomen ◆ Facilitates deep, relaxed breathing ◆ Releases tension in the spine

Partner Two

Massages the stomach, trims the waist, tones the pelvic and abdominal organs ◆ Increases blood-flow to the brain and calms the mind ◆ Stretches the backs of the legs, especially the hamstrings

Standing Double Twist

The Standing Double Twist is unique in that the pose combines a counterbalance with a standing spinal twist. This is a great pose for opening the chest and maintaining a healthy back.

TECHNIQUE

◆ Stand back to back with your partner, open your feet about 4 feet apart, and stretch your arms out to your sides. Cross arms with your partner. Partner One, look to your right. Partner Two, look to your left.

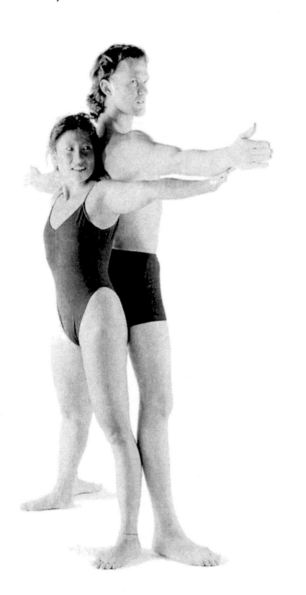

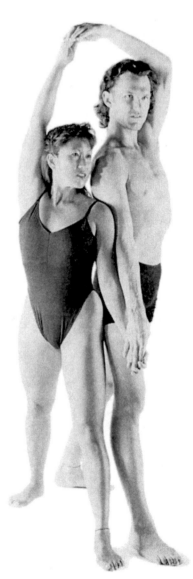

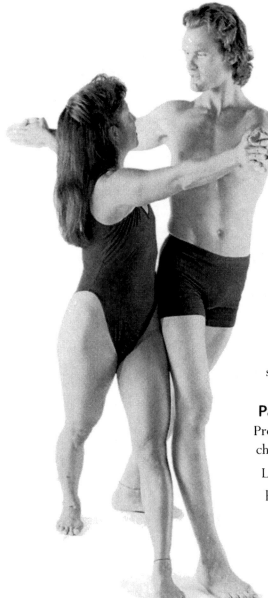

◆ Partner One, turn your right foot to point toward your right side. Partner Two, turn your left foot to point toward your left side.

◆ Both partners, lower your inside arm and raise your outer arm overhead, keeping hand contact at all times. Partner One, begin turning to your right as Two turns to her left.

◆ Maintaining hip contact, complete your turn and open your chests toward each other. This will create a twist at your waist and upper body.

◆ Adjust your hand position so you are palm to palm with your partner.

◆ Breathe, lift your sternum, and relax your shoulders. Hold for 30 to 60 seconds to allow your spine to relax fully.

◆ Slowly release and repeat the pose on the opposite side.

Partner Pointers

Press into your partner at the hips and away at the chest.

Lift your sternum and drop your tailbone to support proper spinal alignment.

Engage your thigh muscles and draw your kneecaps up; this will protect your knees and stabilize the pose.

Relax your shoulders, lengthen your arms, and reach all the way through your fingertips.

CAUTIONS: It is best not to perform twists if you have acute stomach or abdominal problems or hernias, or if you have had recent abdominal surgery. During pregnancy, most twists are not suggested. Gentle twists can be done with utmost care.

Benefits

Relieves stiffness in the neck and shoulders ◆ Stimulates the kidneys and abdominal organs ◆ Improves digestion ◆ Increases flexibility of spine and hips ◆ Relieves backaches and headaches

Double Triangle

The triangle is considered a sacred geometric form in many spiritual traditions. In the Double Triangle pose, two bodies create a series of triangles, which serve to heat the body and ignite the spirit.

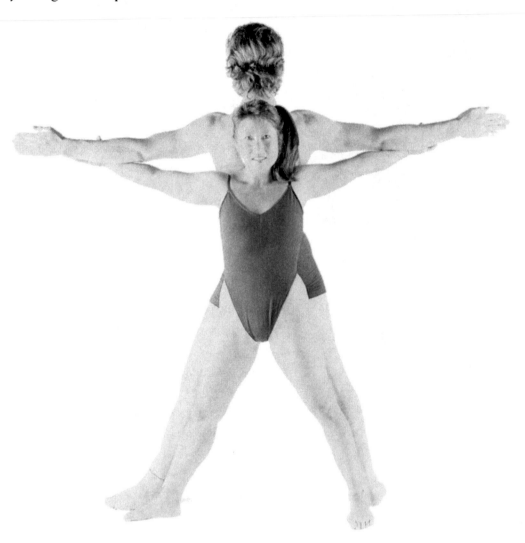

TECHNIQUE

• Stand back to back with your partner and open your feet about 3 to 4 feet apart.

• Touch hands, wrists, or forearms, depending on your different arm lengths, and raise your arms out to your sides, parallel to the ground.

• Point your foot in the direction you are about to bend. Relax your shoulders and breathe.

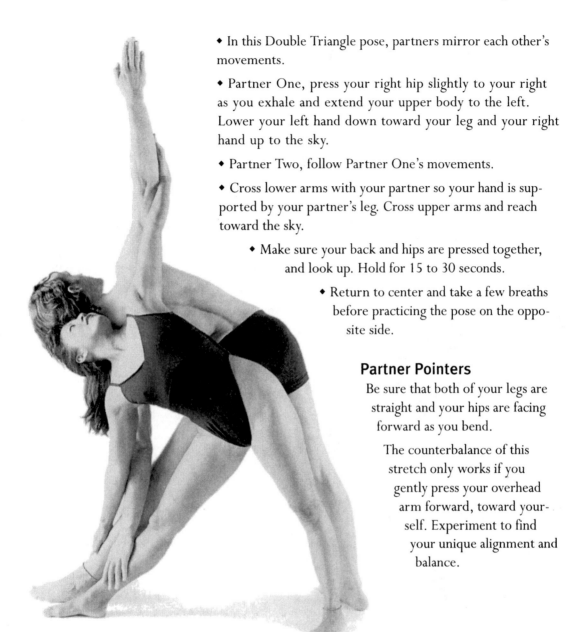

- In this Double Triangle pose, partners mirror each other's movements.

- Partner One, press your right hip slightly to your right as you exhale and extend your upper body to the left. Lower your left hand down toward your leg and your right hand up to the sky.

- Partner Two, follow Partner One's movements.

- Cross lower arms with your partner so your hand is supported by your partner's leg. Cross upper arms and reach toward the sky.

- Make sure your back and hips are pressed together, and look up. Hold for 15 to 30 seconds.

- Return to center and take a few breaths before practicing the pose on the opposite side.

Partner Pointers

Be sure that both of your legs are straight and your hips are facing forward as you bend.

The counterbalance of this stretch only works if you gently press your overhead arm forward, toward yourself. Experiment to find your unique alignment and balance.

NOTE: Your partner's back helps you stay aligned. If you were to imagine sheets of rice paper in front of and behind you, your partner would serve as the rice paper behind you. Only bend as far down as you can without popping your hips forward or back through the imaginary rice paper.

Benefits

Lengthens and invigorates the entire body ◆ Tonifies spinal nerves ◆ Improves digestion and stimulates the kidneys and adrenal glands

Double Revolved Triangle

This pose is a variation of *Parivritta Trikonasana*, which means "revolved triangle." In this pose, the upper body revolves a full 180 degrees, creating a powerful twist that opens the chest and improves the elasticity of the spine.

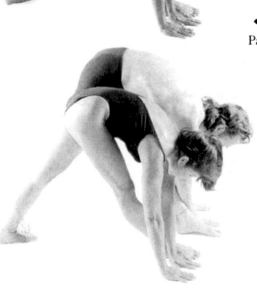

TECHNIQUE

◆ Face your partner, with your toes a couple of inches from your partner's toes and your feet spread 3 to 4 feet.

◆ Partner Two, turn your right foot out at a 90-degree angle.

◆ Inhale and twist your body to the right so your pelvis, navel, and sternum all face directly to the right.

◆ Exhale as you bend your body forward over your right leg.

◆ Place both of your hands on the ground, just to the right of your right foot.

◆ Partner One, assume the same position as Partner Two, except on your left side, so both of you are now facing the same direction.

◆ Partner Two, move the left side of your body down toward your right foot, leaving your left hand down on the ground. Partner One, do the same toward the opposite side.

◆ Partner Two, reach up with your right hand. Partner One, reach up with your left hand to meet Two's hand or arm, depending on your height difference and arm length.

◆ Both partners, look up as you press down with the hand that is on the ground. Cross upper hands or arms, using your partner's counterpressure to increase your stretch.

◆ Hold for 5 to 20 seconds. Breathe smooth and deep.

◆ Return slowly to center and take a few breaths before continuing on the opposite side.

Partner Pointers

Leaning gently into your partner will help you stay balanced. Always stay aware of the balance of the whole pose.

Focus on widening across your chest and back, creating more space between your shoulder blades.

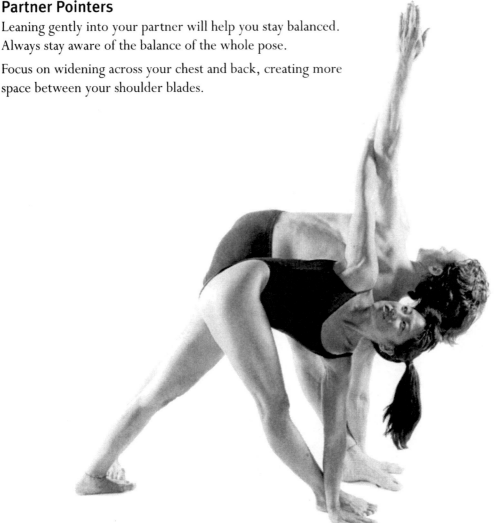

NOTE: Getting a full twist and staying balanced takes practice. Modify the position of your grounded hand if you are unable to make the complete twist, and work into the full posture slowly. You can put your hand on the inner side of your front foot, use a prop such as a wood block, or rest your hand on your leg. Use your partner's back and hips to help you stay aligned and prevent you from swaying your own hips back or front.

CAUTIONS: Don't practice twists if you have acute stomach or abdominal problems or hernias, or if you have had recent abdominal surgery. During pregnancy, this twist is not suggested. Other gentler twists can be done with utmost care.

Benefits

Tones and lengthens the sides of the body ◆ Improves digestion and stimulates the kidneys ◆ Tonifies leg and hip muscles and strengthens ankles ◆ Opens back, chest, and shoulders

The Porthole

The Porthole is a variation of the more traditional Crescent Moon pose. This pose is great for stretching the muscles of the hips and abdomen, namely the psoas and hip flexors.

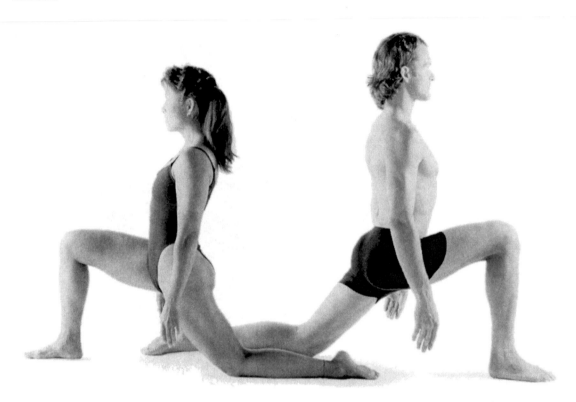

TECHNIQUE

* Stand back to back with your right leg forward and your left leg back about 3 feet. Step forward with your right leg, bending into a lunge until your knee is aligned over your ankle.

* Gently bring your left knee down to the ground. Support yourself with your hands if you are not able to bring your knee down softly. Relax your left leg and position the top of your foot on the ground.

* Inhale, find your balance, and let your hips sink toward the ground, stretching your inner thighs as you exhale.

♦ Inhale, lengthen your spine, then exhale as you begin to lean back, bringing the top of your head or your forehead to meet the top of your partner's head or forehead and reaching your arms overhead.

♦ Hold this posture for 30 to 60 seconds, reaching farther back with your hands as you relax deeper into the stretch. Return to center and switch legs.

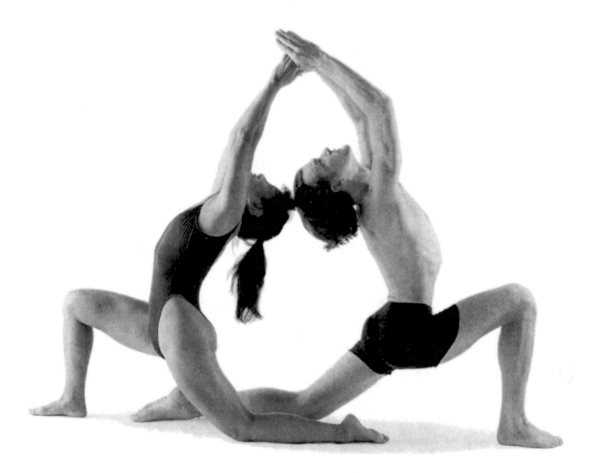

Partner Pointers

Always keep the bent knee over the ankle for maximum stability and minimum strain.

To create a deeper stretch, relax your hips down and forward as you raise your arms overhead.

Benefits

Opens the chest and heart, facilitating deep breathing ♦ Works on alignment and balance
♦ Stretches the thighs and pelvic area ♦ Increases flexibility of the back and shoulders

Double Warrior A

This powerful pose, traditionally known as *Virabhadrasana I*, fills the body with great vigor and strength. This pose helps to keep the whole body supple, yet strong, an aspiration for all great warriors.

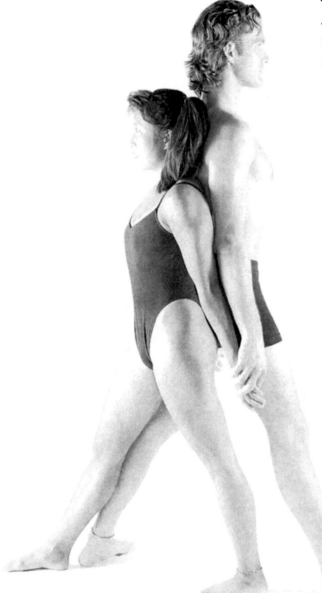

TECHNIQUE

• Begin back to back with your right leg forward and your left leg back about 3 feet.

• Both partners, step forward with your right foot. Keep your back knee as straight as possible (without locking the knee), with your heel reaching toward the ground.

• Lunge forward until your right knee is just over your ankle and your shin is perpendicular to the ground.

• With a deep inhale, reach your arms overhead (behind your ears if possible to give a maximum stretch to your shoulders) and make contact with your partner's hands, wrists, or forearms.

• Exhale and normalize your breathing as you hold the posture for 20 to 40 seconds.

Partner Pointers

Keep pressing your left heel toward the ground and deepening your lunge.

To maintain proper spinal alignment and balance, tuck your tailbone and extend your back leg.

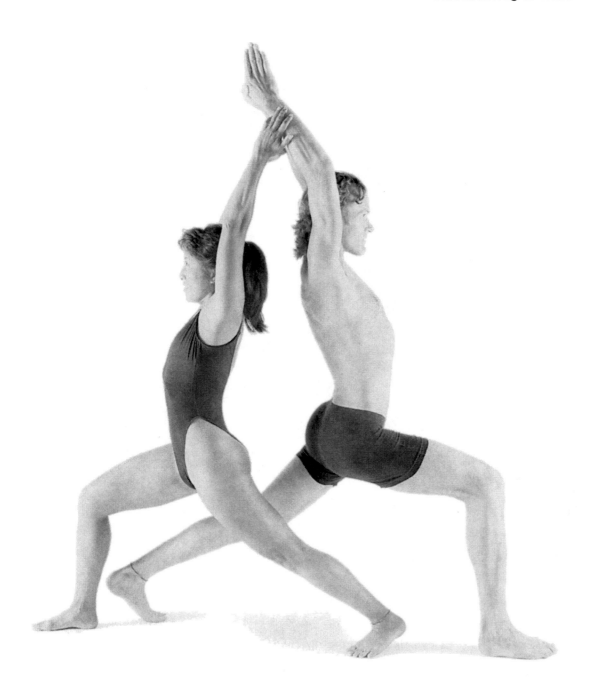

Benefits

Strengthens the legs, especially the thighs ◆ Opens the hips and pelvis ◆ Opens the chest and shoulders ◆ Develops willpower and focus

Rising Cobra

The Cobra or Serpent pose, *Bhujangasana*, is so named because the posture resembles the graceful arch of a cobra's neck as it raises its head. Like a cobra's strike, this dynamic partner pose moves powerful energy up the spine.

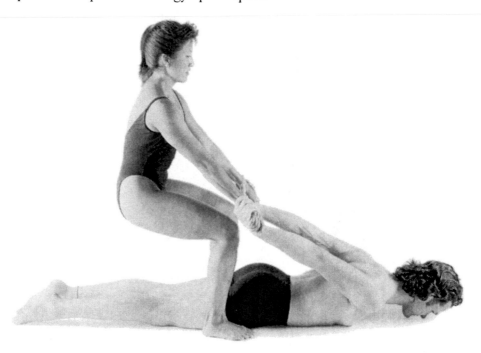

TECHNIQUE

• Partner One, lie face down with your legs together and your hands at your sides.

• Partner Two, stand over One with your feet parallel to his legs, at about the level of his hips or his buttocks.

• Partner Two, bend your knees and take hold of One's wrists. Form a firm yet comfortable hold as you begin to gently lift his arms up.

• Partner One, relax your shoulders and lengthen your spine.

• Partner Two, slowly begin to stand up, assisting One in lifting his torso off the ground. Let him do most of the lifting himself, as this serves to strengthen the lower-back muscles. You are there simply to support him in his stretch.

• Partner Two, tuck your tailbone, press your hips forward, and gently arch back.

• Partner One, tuck your tailbone, press your hips into the floor, and lengthen through your spine.

• Breathe and hold for 10 to 30 seconds. Come out of the pose slowly and rest, lying face down, before switching positions.

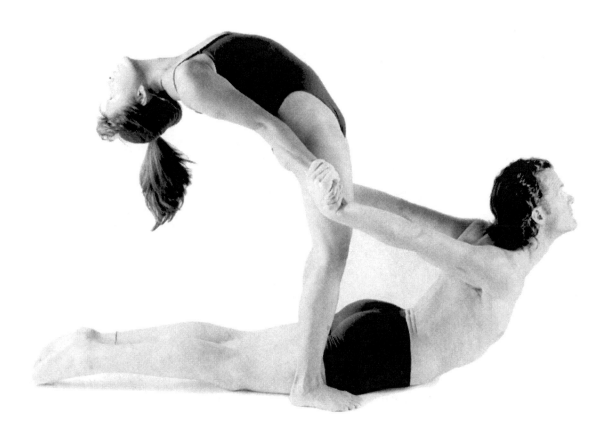

Partner Pointers

Keep your neck in natural alignment with the rest of your spine. Dropping your head back or holding it up causes tension and strain.

Adjust the position of Two's feet so that both partners can comfortably straighten their arms when stretching back.

NOTE: To protect your spine, it is important to flex your buttocks and tuck your tailbone. Always lengthen through your entire spine.

CAUTIONS: Always warm up thoroughly before practicing a back bend. Back-bending postures are not recommended for those with high blood pressure or a history of stroke. Back bending is not recommended for those with acute spinal or neck injuries.

Benefits

Tonifies entire spine and increases flexibility ◆ Opens the chest, abdomen, and shoulders ◆ Strengthens back and butt muscles ◆ Eases menstrual and digestive irregularities

Double Boat

This is the partner variation of *Navasana*, the Boat Pose. The Double Boat is great for stretching the hamstrings and toning the abdomen.

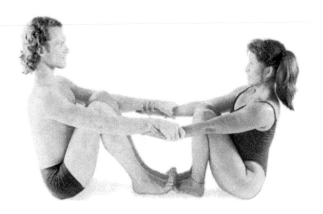 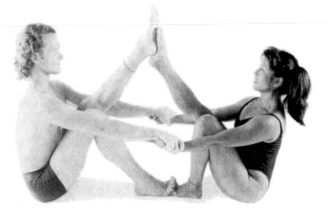

TECHNIQUE

◆ Sit facing your partner, knees pulled in, feet flat on the ground and toes pointed up, touching the bottoms of your partner's toes. Reach forward and link hands or wrists.

◆ Inhale and lengthen your spine. Using the counterpressure from your partner's foot, exhale and straighten one leg, lifting your feet up toward the sky.

◆ Hold for a few breaths to find your balance.

◆ Now lift and straighten your other leg using the same technique.

◆ Keep your arms parallel to the ground and your backs lengthened. Lift from your chest and relax your abdomen.

◆ Breathe deeply and hold for 15 to 30 seconds. Release the pose slowly, one leg at a time.

Partner Pointers

Adjust the distance between you and your partner to find the angle that works best for you.

Focus on lifting from the sternum and opening the chest area, while keeping your shoulders relaxed.

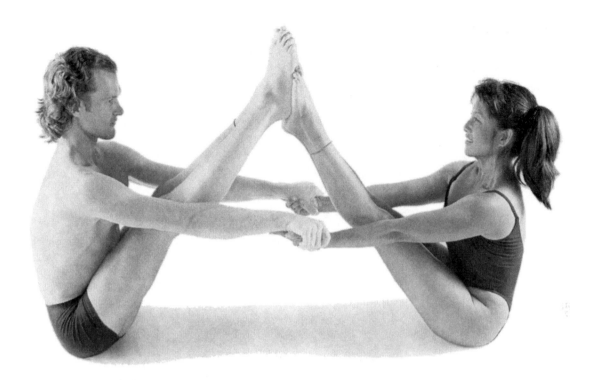

VARIATION: If you find it difficult to straighten your legs completely, practice the variation shown below. Begin sitting a little farther apart than in the original Double Boat beginning posture.

Instead of straightening your legs fully, bring one leg up and keep it bent. Then bring the other leg up and keep both bent.

Use the pressure from your partner's feet and the pull from her hands to help you press your thighs into your chest and lengthen your spine.

Balance, breathe, and hold for 15 to 30 seconds. Release slowly, one leg at a time.

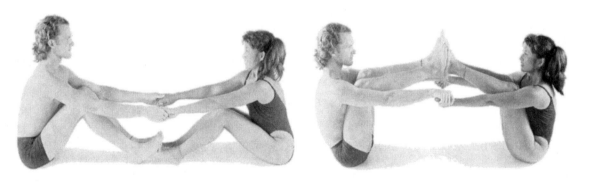

Benefits

Strengthens abdominal muscles ◆ Improves digestion ◆ Tonifies kidneys ◆ Stretches the backs of legs

Double Straddle

Double Straddle is a heart-connecting pose. This intense leg stretch is a variation of *Upavista Konasana*, which means Seated Angle Pose.

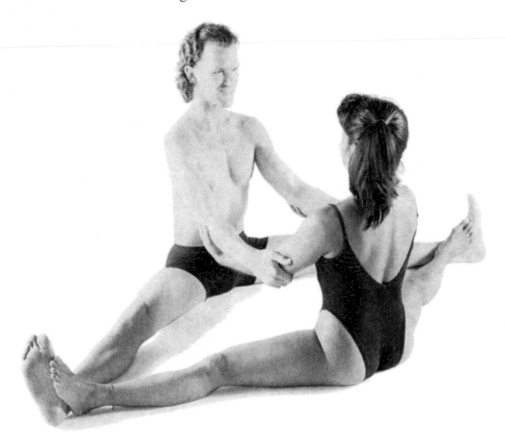

TECHNIQUE

♦ Sit facing your partner with your legs open in a straddle position. Keep your knees and toes facing up.

♦ Press your feet against your partner's feet. Use your partner's feet to keep your toes pointing up and even slightly back. This will increase your inner thigh stretch.

♦ Touch hands or arms, smile, and breathe gently with your partner.

♦ As you feel comfortable, increase your stretch by scooting slowly toward your partner and pressing your feet farther out to the sides. If you can, move close enough to your partner to release your handhold and reach for the backs of his legs.

♦ Press the backs of your knees toward the ground, lengthen your spine, and breathe.

♦ Hold for 30 to 60 seconds and come out of the posture slowly.

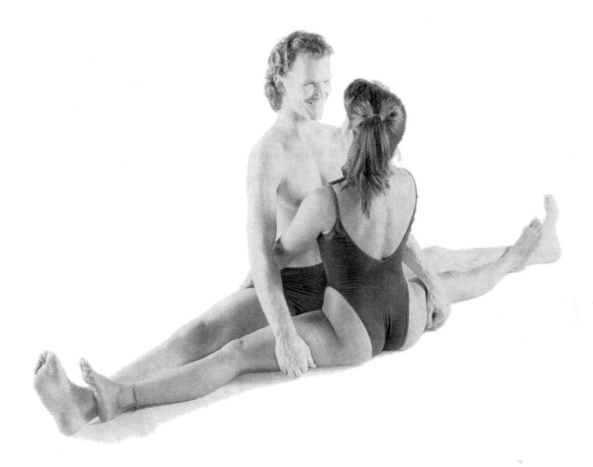

Partner Pointers

Press your sitz bones into the floor and reach your sternum and head up to the sky.

You may need to support yourself with your hands on the ground behind you as you widen your straddle. Once you're comfortable, resume holding your partner's arms or legs.

CAUTIONS: Do not pull on your partner's legs. Move deeper into the pose by breathing, relaxing, and using your hands to lightly encourage the stretch.

Benefits

Increases hip and inner-thigh flexibility ◆ Tonifies leg muscles ◆ Increases blood circulation to the pelvic organs ◆ Especially good for gynecological problems, for menstrual irregularities, and during pregnancy

Spinal Twist 1 and 2

This Spinal Twist called *Ardha Matsyendrasana* gets its name from the great sage *Matsyendra*. This pose helps to relieve tension in the lower back while deeply massaging the abdominal organs.

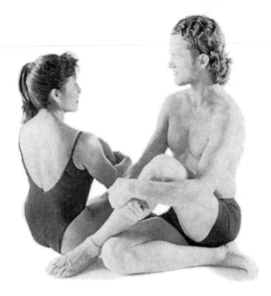

TECHNIQUE

- Sit side by side, facing the opposite direction of your partner.

- Partner One, sit on your right buttock and cross your left leg over your right.

- Wrap your arms around your left leg and pull up on your bent knee so it points toward the sky.

- Leave your left foot on the ground as you sit down. Settle your buttocks on the floor.

- Partner Two, do the same.

- Both, look at your partner, breathe deeply, and lengthen your spine.

- Exhale as you begin to twist toward your left. Bring your left arm behind your back and extend your right arm forward to connect with your partner's hand behind her back.

- Complete the twist by looking over your left shoulder. Increase the stretch by reaching farther up your partner's arm.

- Hold for 30 to 60 seconds, release slowly, and change sides.

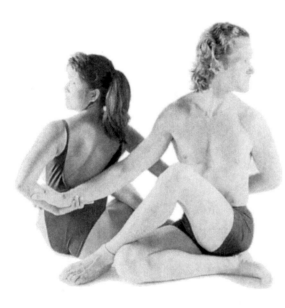

- For Spinal Twist 2, assume the same starting position. To increase the stretch, reach your right arm to the outside of your left knee.

- Now reach back with your left arm for your partner's hand. As you press your right arm on your left knee, you will increase the stretch.

- Exhale, look over your left shoulder, and twist a little farther to your left. Continue lengthening your spine.

- Hold for 30 to 60 seconds, release slowly, and change sides.

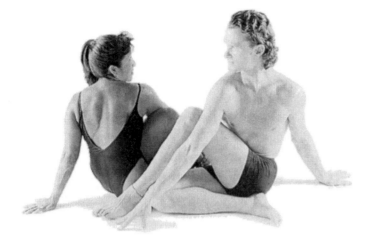

Partner Pointers

Breathe deeply into your abdomen, as this stimulates and massages your abdominal organs.

Keep your shoulders level and relaxed.

Press both your sitz bones toward the ground as you twist. It is best to keep your right foot close to your hip. If sitting this way causes strain on your right knee, however, leave your right leg extended straight.

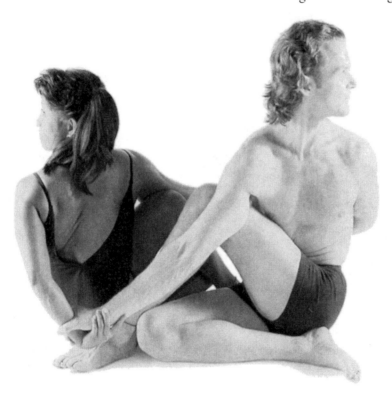

CAUTIONS: Do not practice these poses if you are pregnant, have abdominal problems or a hernia, or have had recent abdominal surgery.

Benefits

Increases spinal flexibility ◆ Stretches and strengthens external and internal oblique muscles ◆ Tonifies spinal nerves and ligaments ◆ Stimulates digestion and all abdominal organs

Two Scoops 1 and 2

Two Scoops was so named because the pose looks like a double scoop of ice cream. This is a playful pose that challenges your balance and concentration.

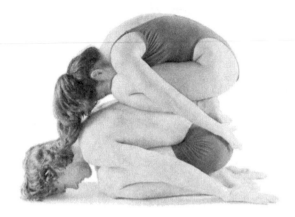

TECHNIQUE

• Partner One, move into Child Pose.

• Partner Two, climb onto Partner One's back with your knees. Find just the perfect place for your knees on One's back.

• Partner Two, inhale and find your balance. Exhale, bend forward into Child Pose, and relax your arms behind you, palms facing up.

• Hold for 30 to 60 seconds and then switch places.

• Both partners, place your hands under your forehead for a slight variation to Two Scoops 1. We call this Two Scoops 2.

Partner Pointers

It may take a few attempts to find your balance in this pose. Play with the posture and remember that wobbling is half the fun.

If you're the top scoop and you need to stabilize yourself, hold on to your partner's back until you feel comfortable enough to let go.

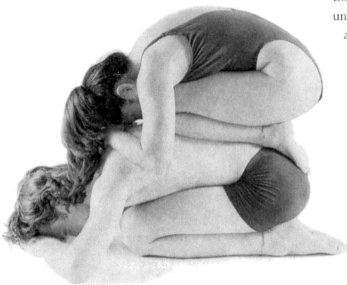

Benefits

Works on balancing as a team ◆ Relaxes the body, calms the mind, and normalizes circulation ◆ Counter-stretches the spine after any backward bend

Partner Plow

A great yogi once said, "Sow love, reap peace . . . sow meditation, reap wisdom." The Partner Plow is used for this very purpose.

TECHNIQUE

◆ Place a folded towel or blanket on the floor.

◆ Partner One, lie on your back with your shoulders and upper arms on the blanket and your head resting on the floor. Bring your legs together and place your hands at your sides, palms down.

◆ Partner One, inhale, bend your knees, and raise your hips off the ground. Bend your elbows and support your back as you raise your hips.

◆ Partner One, exhale and gently lift your legs over your head, keeping your knees bent. Lower your feet to the ground over your head and straighten your legs.

◆ Partner One, bring your arms down to the ground behind you.

◆ Partner Two, press up against One's back, inhaling and lengthening your spine. Bring One's arms as close to your legs as possible.

◆ Hold for 15 to 45 seconds and release slowly. Rest on your back before switching positions with your partner.

Partner Pointers

Partner One, always be mindful of the position of your chin, and be careful that you are not flattening the cervical curve in your neck.

Partner One, closing your eyes keeps your mind relaxed and focused.

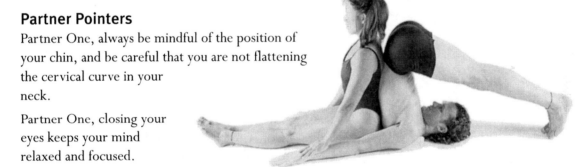

CAUTIONS: Do not practice Plow if you have neck or back injuries. Be careful not to press your chin into your throat. This will flatten your cervical curve. Relax your neck and allow your chin to rest naturally toward your chest in the space between your collarbones. Inversions are not suggested when menstruating.

Benefits

Partner One
> Increases circulation to the brain ◆ Normalizes the thyroid gland ◆ Releases tension in the spine

Partner Two
> Increases awareness of alignment ◆ Stretches the back of the legs ◆ Gives you time to relax and connect with being a supportive partner

Partner Shoulderstand

The Shoulderstand is one of the most rejuvenating and invigorating of all of the yoga poses. In fact, this pose is known as the mother of all asanas and is said to stimulate every cell of the body.

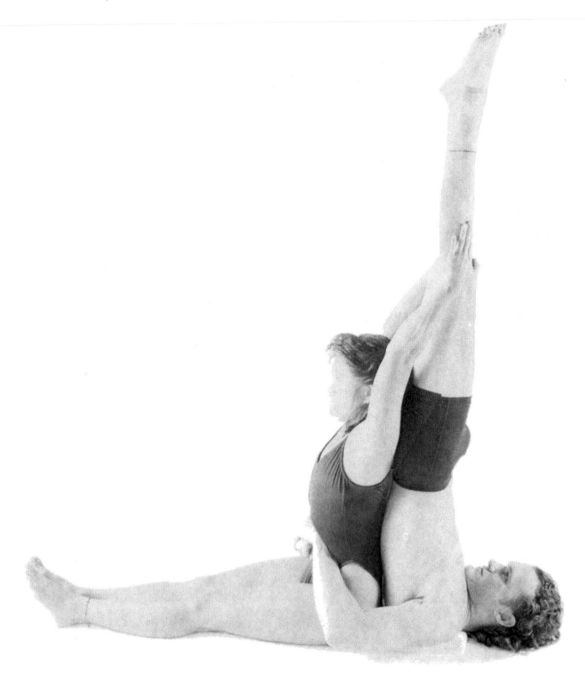

TECHNIQUE

• This pose is an extension of Partner Plow (see page 123). Move into the posture just as if you were getting into Partner Plow.

• Partner One, from the Plow position, raise your legs with your toes pointing straight up to the sky. Use Two's counterpressure along with your abdominal muscles to help you lift into the shoulderstand. Then reach your arms around Two's waist.

• Partner Two, reach up with your arms and hold One's legs. As you stretch up, gently traction One's legs up to increase his stretch as well as lengthen your spine.

• Hold for 30 seconds to a few minutes, and then release the posture very slowly and rest lying on your back in Corpse Pose (see page 65) for a few breaths. Switch positions with your partner.

Partner Pointers

Partner One, do not jerk when coming up into the shoulderstand. Lift your legs up slowly using your abdominal muscles or your arms for support.

Partner One, use your partner's back for support, as this allows you to increase your stretch while maintaining stability.

Partner One, point your toes up, yet keep them relaxed. Tension anywhere in the body leads to strain.

Partner One, rest as little weight as possible on your neck; most of the weight is on your shoulders. When lifting your legs, bend your knees if you need to. Otherwise, keep your legs straight and work your abdominal muscles. When Two moves away from your back and you are releasing the pose, use your hands on your lower back or hips for support. Alternate between Shoulderstand and Partner Plow to strengthen your abdominal muscles.

CAUTIONS: Do not practice Partner Shoulderstand if you have neck or back injuries. Be careful not to press your chin into your throat. This will flatten your cervical curve. Relax your neck and allow it to come naturally to your chest in the space between your collarbones. Inversions are not suggested when menstruating.

Benefits

Partner One
> Stimulates the thyroid and parathyroid glands ◆ Increases flexibility of the spine, especially the neck ◆ Encourages deep abdominal breathing ◆ Increases circulation, which is especially good for varicose veins or tired, aching legs

Partner Two
> Allows time for you to focus on your alignment ◆ Stretches the spine ◆ Gives you time to relax and connect with being a supportive partner

Child Camel

This relaxing posture allows for mutual support while moving deeper into an exploration of trust and surrender.

TECHNIQUE

- Partner One, kneel and sit back on your feet in a relaxed position.

- Partner Two, kneel, placing your back against Partner One and your lower legs and feet on the ground outside of One's legs.

- Both, lengthen through your spine and breathe.

- Partner One, bend forward into Child Pose, bringing your upper body over your thighs. Rest your forehead on the ground.

- Partner Two, as One bends forward, exhale and lean over his back, moving down into a supported back arch. Inhale, reach overhead with your arms, and gently cradle One's forehead in your hands.

- Hold the pose for 30 to 60 seconds, breathing normally. Come back to center and rest before reversing roles.

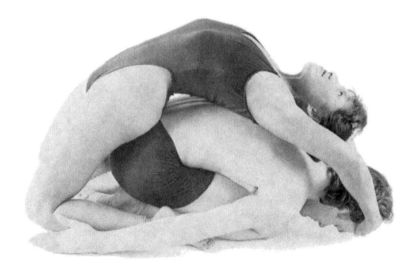

Partner Pointers

When coming up from the back bend, lead from your chest rather than lifting your head up and straining your neck. First release the posture, then allow your neck to relax and your head to naturally return to the upright position.

Pay attention to areas of your back that are stiffer, and work on developing an even extension of your spine.

If the ground is hard on your knees, kneel on a towel or blanket.

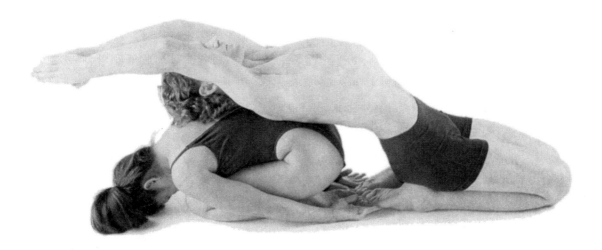

VARIATION: If one of you is much taller than the other, begin farther away from your partner's back. Partner One, start toe-to-toe (or farther or closer depending on the height difference) instead of bringing your legs to the outside of your partner's legs. Support yourself bending back as you gently lean on your partner's back. Then release your arms overhead for the final stretch.

CAUTIONS: Always warm up thoroughly before practicing a back bend. Back-bending postures are not recommended for those with high blood pressure or a history of stroke. Back bending is not recommended for those with spinal or neck injuries.

Benefits

Partner One

Child Pose relaxes the mind and normalizes breathing ◆ Counter-stretches the spine after any backward bend ◆ Allows you to feel safe and protected

Partner Two

Allows you to safely open deeper into your back bend ◆ Irrigates the spinal discs ◆ Stretches the shoulders and opens the chest

Heart Opener

The Heart Opener is so named because you expand your chest and give your heart maximum space to open. It is a combination of Child Pose with a variation of the traditional fish pose, *Matsyasana*, named after a Hindu god who turned himself into a fish to save the world from a flood. The person in Child Pose goes inward and creates a stable base. With this strong foundation, her partner can feel safe enough to become vulnerable and open his heart.

TECHNIQUE

• Partner One, sit with your spine lengthened and your legs straight out in front of you.

• Partner Two, kneel back to back with Partner One.

• Both partners, lengthen your spine, breathe, and relax.

• Partner Two, bend forward into Child Pose.

• Partner One, exhale and lie gently on Two's back, leaving your legs together or bringing them a foot or two apart.

• Both partners, stretch your arms out to your sides and bring your hands together.

• Partner Two, using the weight of gravity, gently press One's arms toward the floor. Breathe deeply together, holding the posture for up to a minute or two.

• Return to center for a few breaths before switching positions.

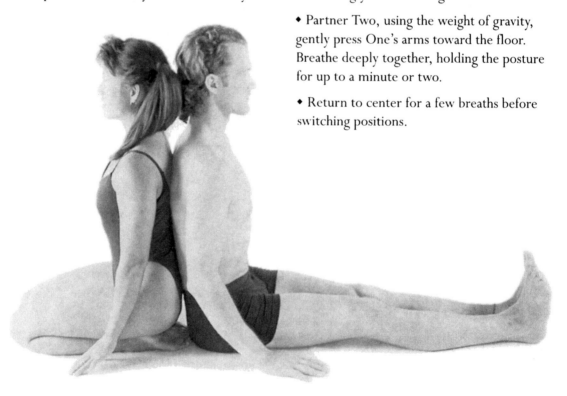

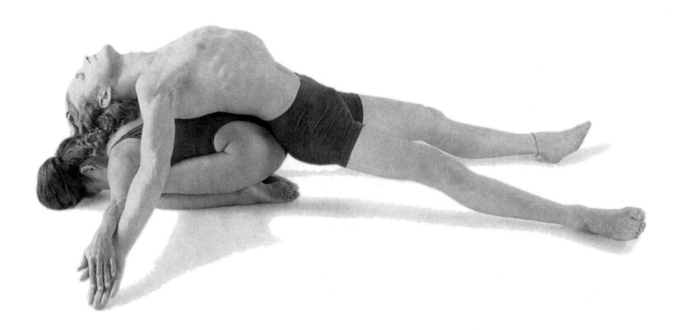

Partner Pointers

Partner One, maintain length in your spine by lifting through your sternum and allowing your tail-bone to drop.

Partner One, widen through your back and allow your chest and ribs to become supple as you breathe.

Partner Two, maintain smooth and even breathing.

Partner Two, focus on feeling the connection between your back and your partner's back.

Benefits

Partner One

Provides an excellent counter-stretch to the Plow and Shoulderstand ◆ Relieves stiffness and tension in the neck and shoulders ◆ Opens the chest, expands the rib cage, and deepens breathing ◆ Creates space around the heart and a sense of peace

Partner Two

Allows you time to rest and rejuvenate ◆ Counter-stretches the spine after any back bend ◆ Stimulates the abdominal organs ◆ Brings blood to the brain and relieves mental fatigue

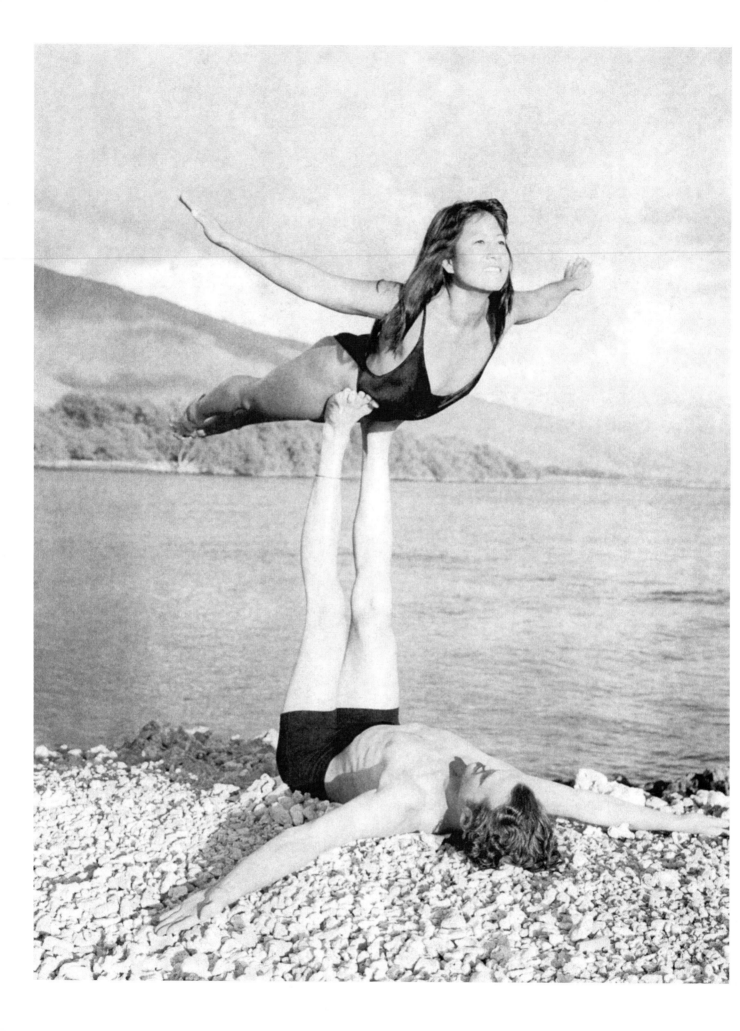

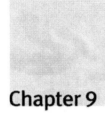

Chapter 9

Balancing on the Graceful Edge

"When the strings of your lute were neither too taut nor too loose, but adjusted to an even pitch, did your lute then have a wonderful sound and was it easily playable? If energy is applied too strong, it will lead to restlessness, and if energy is too lax, it will lead to lassitude. Therefore, keep your energy in balance and in this way focus your attention."

—Anguttara Nikaya, *Parable of the Lute, Teachings of Buddha*

From a strong underground foundation, trees reach up from the earth to touch the sky and embrace the sun. Their heavy branches stretch forth in all directions, and their balance and grace seem almost effortless. Even in the midst of whirling storms and changing seasons, trees remain poised and ever present. As humans, many of us spend our entire lives striving for what trees seem to embody inherently. Instead of simply living in the moment, we exhaust ourselves running in circles like cats chasing their tails. The truth is, within each of us there is a place of perfect balance that can be realized only when we stop trying so hard. This place of balance can be found in the present moment, sometimes hidden between our fears and our self-imposed limitations. It takes courage to arrive there, and when we do, we are closest to our true nature.

In chapter 7, you practiced postures for strength, stamina, and flexibility. In chapter 8, you moved a bit deeper and experienced postures that require trust and surrender. Now, in chapter 9, we invite you to explore some of the most challenging postures in Partner Yoga. As you practice these postures, work with your partner to move consciously toward the edge of your fears and limitations. Stay present with each pose and immerse yourself in the total experience.

The most advanced postures are the lifts, beginning on page 148. In practicing a single partner lift posture, you capture the essence of the Partner Yoga experience—total cooperation, complete trust, and absolute commitment to the present moment. The lifts challenge your strength, balance, and focus, and they bring you face to face with your fears. In return, the lift postures bring you closer to your true self and leave you with an exhilarating sense of freedom.

For some of you, these postures will push you to the edge of your physical ability. For others, the challenge may be more mental, emotional, or spiritual. Either way, the key is to find the courage to stand your ground in the face of that which daunts you. Your partner is there to support you, yet as you continue farther on this journey, there will come a time when the road narrows and each of you will have to proceed alone; for only you know the way to your true self. Perhaps spiritual leader Sathya Sai Baba says it best when he writes, "Life is a pilgrimage where man drags his feet along the rough and thorny road. . . . There is no stopping place in this pilgrimage. . . . When the road ends, and the Goal is gained, the pilgrim finds that he traveled only from himself to himself."

CAUTIONS

Lifts are risky poses. We strongly advise that you always practice lifts with reverence and utmost care. Also, practice lifts in a clear, open space where you can fall without injuring yourself. Falling is part of the learning process. Support each other in making landings as soft as possible. The base partner may want to use a thin pad under the sacrum and lower back while practicing lifts (a sticky mat or thin towel works best). In addition, lifted postures are not recommended for those with high blood pressure, history of stroke, or acute spinal or neck injuries, or for women who are pregnant. Inverted lifts (where the pelvis is higher than the head) are not recommended for women who are menstruating.

Double Tree

In an ever-changing world, we each need to find our center of balance and power. The Tree Pose, *Vriksasana*, is a hatha yoga standard that will help you to do just that.

TECHNIQUE

- Stand hip to hip with your foot about 10 inches from your partner's.

- Reach your arm around your partner's waist and create a firm connection between your hips. Lift your outside leg and place your foot against the upper part of your opposing inner thigh.

- Join the palm of your free hand together with your partner's at center. Breathe.

- Hold the pose for 15 to 30 seconds. Repeat on the other side.

Partner Pointers

Each partner must first find his own balance, bringing balance into the partnership. The pose is based on mutual support, not one partner holding the other up.

Become acutely aware of your standing leg and foot. Feel how your standing foot roots you to the ground and how your body raises up and balances over that strong base.

VARIATION: For a more expansive pose and a slightly more challenging balance, try the variation shown to the left. From the Double Tree, slowly lift your hand from around your partner's waist while keeping your hip pressed firmly together with your partner's. Raise your arm straight up while pulling gently in on your partner's arm toward the center. Inhale, and raise your free arm parallel to the floor. Relax your shoulders and expand through your chest. Breathe.

Benefits

Tones muscles of the hips, legs, and feet ◆ Improves balance and posture ◆ Focuses the mind and creates calm in the face of challenge

Standing Star

Traditionally this pose is called *Utthita Hasta Padangusthasana*, which literally means extended (*utthita*) hand (*hasta*) to foot (*pada*) pose (*asana*). Although we do have a fondness for Sanskrit, we prefer to call this balancing pose the Standing Star.

TECHNIQUE

◆ Stand hip to hip with your inner foot about 10 inches from your partner's. Reach your arm around your partner's waist and create a firm connection between your hips.

◆ Lift your outside leg and hold the big toe with your forefinger and thumb.

◆ Inhale, and lengthen out through your standing leg and spine.

◆ Exhale. While keeping hold of your big toe, slowly straighten your knee and extend your leg out to the side.

◆ Relax your shoulders and open through your chest and ribs. Breathe.

◆ Hold the pose for 5 to 20 seconds. Repeat on the other side.

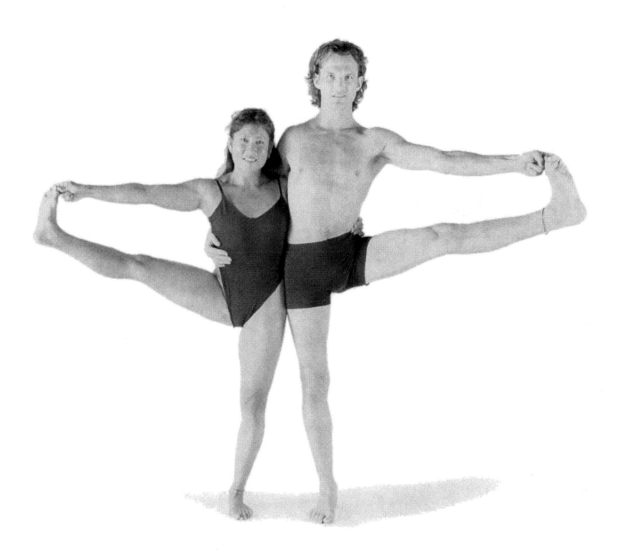

Partner Pointers

As you extend your leg out to the side, send your breath into that leg and out through the heel. Imagine your leg becoming long and light as it fills with breath.

Practice the same visualization with your arm. Send your breath into your extended arm and out through your fingertips, allowing your arm to lengthen and become light.

Benefits

Strengthens leg and hip muscles ◆ Stretches the hamstrings and inner thighs ◆ Develops a strong sense of center and balance ◆ Allows you to feel both grounded and expansive

Reaching for the Moon

This pose couples the Half Moon Pose, *Ardha Chandrasana*, with a reaching back bend, to create an expansive partner pose that develops strength, flexibility, and balance.

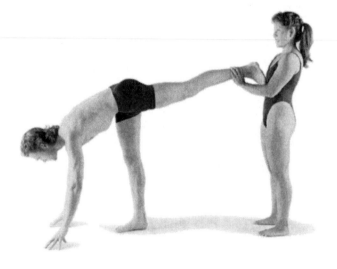

TECHNIQUE

♦ Partner One, start in Mellow Mountain Pose, facing away from your partner. Bend forward from your hips as you lift your left leg behind you. Then lower your hands to the floor in front of you (maintain a slight bend in your standing leg).

♦ Partner Two, quickly squat down and catch One's lifted ankle. Slowly rise up to Mountain Pose, holding One's foot at your chest.

♦ Partner One, bring your right hand in front of your right foot, and begin to rotate your body up so that your left hip rests on top of your right hip (your right arm and leg are parallel about 1 foot apart). Inhale, lift your left arm toward the sky, and lengthen through your chest and back.

♦ Partner Two, make sure One's left foot, knee, hip, and shoulder are all in the same line, and that his standing leg is perpendicular to the floor.

♦ Partner One, exhale and lower your left arm down to your left ear and extend out through your fingertips.

♦ Partner Two, inhale, lengthen out through your spine, and slowly lift One's foot overhead (the height of the foot will depend on One's level of flexibility). Exhale, tuck your tailbone, lift your chest, and arch gently into a back bend.

♦ Breathe smooth and deep. Hold the pose for 5 to 15 seconds. Repeat on the other side.

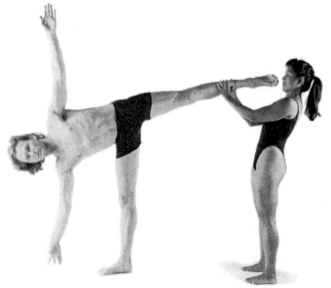

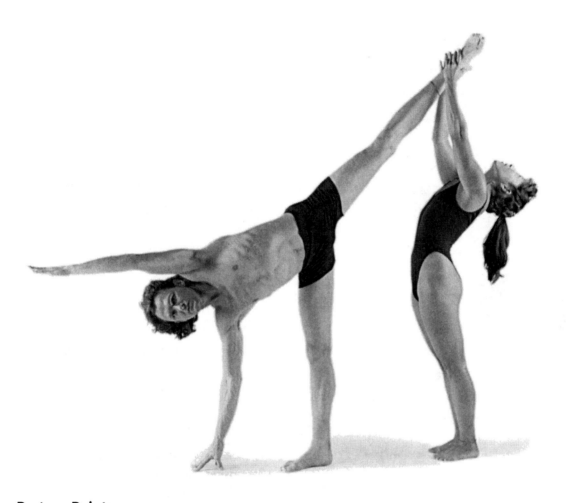

Partner Pointers

Partner One, to develop a powerful Moon Pose, you must first root firmly into the standing leg and supporting hand, then consciously extend the lifted leg and arm in opposite directions, creating a feeling of length and lightness.

Partner Two, keep your movements smooth and stay keenly aware of the balance of the pose as a whole.

Benefits

Partner One
   Strengthens calves, thighs, and buttocks ◆ Increases flexibility in hamstrings and inner-thigh muscles ◆ Opens rib cage and tones the deep abdominal muscles

Partner Two
   Frees the front of the body ◆ Increases range of motion in spine ◆ Increases balance and sensitivity to your partner's alignment

Double Dancer

Natarajasana is the Sanskrit name of this pose. *Nataraja* is the name of Siva, the Cosmic Dancer. Poised and graceful, he symbolizes the eternal cycle of life—creation, preservation, and destruction. In practicing Double Dancer, we catch a glimpse of the cosmic dancer within.

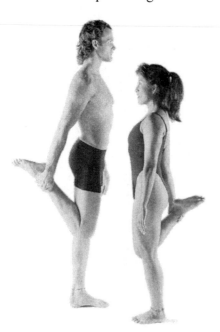

TECHNIQUE

• Stand facing your partner, slightly staggered and about 1 foot apart. Root firmly into your left foot and lift your right foot up behind you, holding your ankle with your right hand.

• Inhale, lengthen your spine, relax your shoulders, and establish your balance. Exhale, lean slowly forward, and reach your left arm up to your partner's right foot.

• Inhale as you lift your right knee and foot toward the sky. Maintain smooth and consistent breathing.

• Hold for 5 to 15 seconds. Repeat on the other side.

Partner Pointers

Remember, each posture in Partner Yoga represents one complete form that two people create. As you practice Double Dancer, stay aware of the balance of the whole pose. Work *with* your partner to create grace and stability.

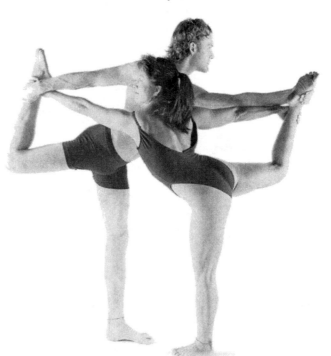

Benefits

Strengthens and stretches hip and thigh muscles ◆ Strengthens your sense of center ◆ Increases awareness of balance and grace ◆ Builds teamwork between partners

The M Bend

The M Bend is a powerful forward bending straddle that stretches the backs of the legs while opening the chest and shoulders.

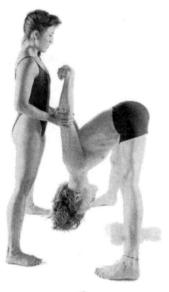

TECHNIQUE

• Partner One, stand with your legs about 3 feet apart. Inhale, lengthen your spine, and clasp your hands behind your back. Exhale, slowly bending forward from your hips and lifting your arms.

• Partner Two, stand in front of One with your legs in the same position. Support One's arms as he bends forward.

• Partner Two, inhale, lengthen your spine, and clasp your hands behind your back. Exhale, slowly bending forward from your hips and lifting your arms until you make contact with your partner's arms (you may need to walk forward or back slightly to find the right position).

• Both partners, hold your arms together at the centerline of the pose and breathe into your ribs and back.

• Hold the pose for 10 to 30 seconds.

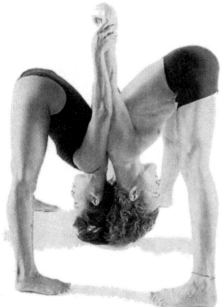

Partner Pointers

As you hang in the forward bend, allow your head and neck to relax. Feel the pull of gravity on your head, and allow this gentle pull to move you deeper into the stretch. Imagine that this downward pull is lengthening your spine, creating more space between each vertebra.

Benefits

Opens the chest, ribs, and shoulders ◆ Stretches the hamstrings, buttocks, and lower back
◆ Increases bloodflow to the brain ◆ Stimulates the digestive organs

Lateral Angle

This pose is a variation of *Utthita Parsvakonasana*, the Extended Lateral Angle Pose. As the name implies, this pose tones and invigorates the sides of the body.

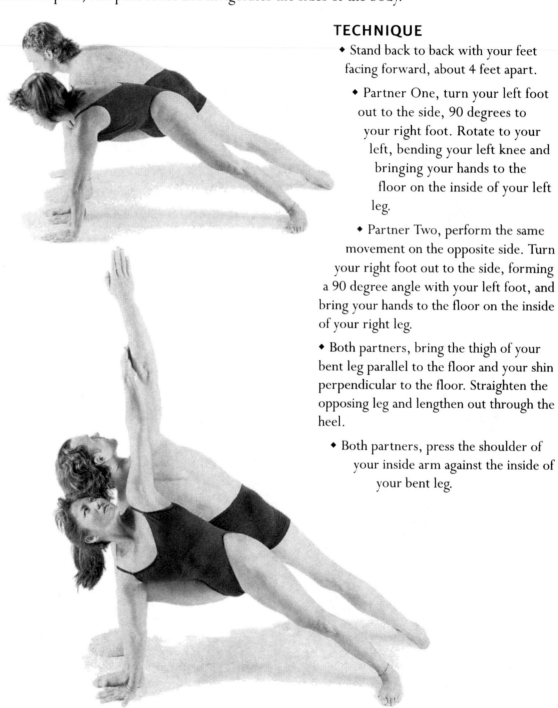

TECHNIQUE

- Stand back to back with your feet facing forward, about 4 feet apart.

- Partner One, turn your left foot out to the side, 90 degrees to your right foot. Rotate to your left, bending your left knee and bringing your hands to the floor on the inside of your left leg.

- Partner Two, perform the same movement on the opposite side. Turn your right foot out to the side, forming a 90 degree angle with your left foot, and bring your hands to the floor on the inside of your right leg.

- Both partners, bring the thigh of your bent leg parallel to the floor and your shin perpendicular to the floor. Straighten the opposing leg and lengthen out through the heel.

- Both partners, press the shoulder of your inside arm against the inside of your bent leg.

◆ Inhale, rotating your torso up and lifting your outside arm toward the sky. Connect hands with your partner as you reach up (pull gently toward yourself to create a counterbalance). Look up toward your up-stretched hand. Exhale, and lower the up-stretched arm down to your ear.

◆ Lengthen your arm forward and extend out through your fingertips. Continue to look up, relaxing your neck and shoulders.

◆ Breathe smooth and deep. Hold the pose for 10 to 20 seconds. Repeat on the other side.

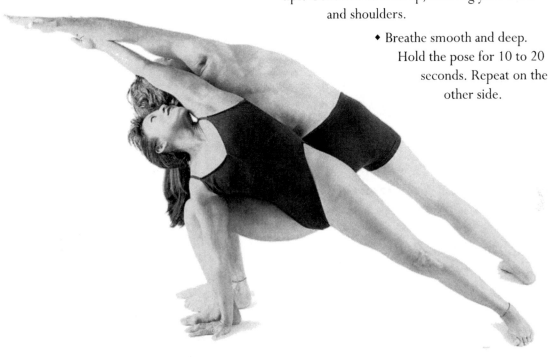

Partner Pointers

Experiment with the distance between you and your partner, and the amount of pull on your upper arm. The key is to find a place where you both feel relaxed and balanced.

Extend through your back leg and reach the outside of your foot into the floor.

Benefits

Releases stuck energy in the pelvic region ◆ Opens the sides of the body (specifically the oblique and intercostal muscles) ◆ Strengthens the thighs and calves ◆ Increases peristaltic activity, aiding digestion, absorption, and elimination

Yin Yang Handstand

When opposites come together, there is yoga, union. So it is with the Yin Yang Handstand.
Partners find harmony within the opposing movements.

TECHNIQUE

◆ Stand facing your partner about 3 feet apart.

◆ Partner Two, lift your hands and get ready to catch One's legs.

◆ Partner One, bring your palms to the floor, about 1 foot in front of Two's feet (your hands are
shoulder-width apart, fingers spread wide). Bend your knees slightly and prepare to kick up into
the handstand.

◆ Partner One, inhale and lengthen out through your arms and shoulders, and root your hands
firmly on the floor. Exhale, and kick up into a handstand.

◆ Partner Two, catch One's legs as they come over, and hold the
legs perpendicular to the floor (more or less parallel to your
body).

◆ Both partners, keep length in your spine and tuck
your tailbone. Breathe deeply.

◆ Hold the pose for 5 to 15 seconds.
Switch roles.

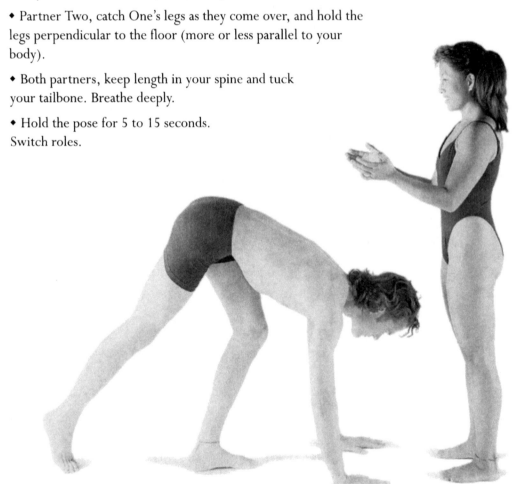

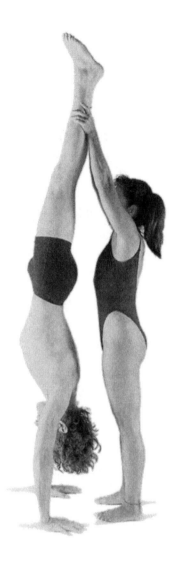

Partner Pointers

It may take a few tries to find the perfect body position. Everyone finds balance and strength in the handstand differently. Communication is essential.

If you find that you don't have the arm and shoulder strength to perform the handstand, practice Double Downward Dog frequently (see page 70). This pose will strengthen your shoulders and arms and prepare your body for the handstand.

Partner One, you have to trust that your partner will catch you as you go into the handstand. You can practice on a wall to get used to the feeling of having support behind you (although a wall is certainly no substitute for your partner).

Partner Two, be sensitive to the possibility of One's fear or hesitation.

CAUTIONS: Handstands are not recommended for those with high blood pressure or a history of stroke, or for women who are pregnant or menstruating.

Benefits

Partner One

Strengthens the arms and shoulders ◆ Increases circulation to the brain and stimulates the pituitary gland ◆ Consistent practice relieves, and possibly reverses, varicose veins ◆ Develops willpower and enthusiasm

Partner Two

Creates an upward flow of energy ◆ Develops good posture ◆ Increases awareness of alignment and weight distribution

Double Scorpion

The Double Scorpion is an advanced inversion that challenges your will and concentration. This is a powerful pose for building upper-body strength and spinal flexibility.

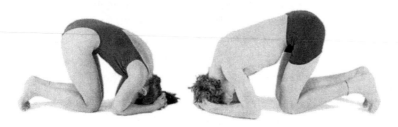

TECHNIQUE

• To work into the Double Scorpion, you must first be able to hold steady and relaxed in the Headstand. Begin by facing your partner on your hands and knees.

• To warm up your neck, rock your head forward and back and from side to side.

• Place your elbows under your shoulders and your palms flat on the floor (adjust your position so that your fingertips are a couple of inches from your partner's).

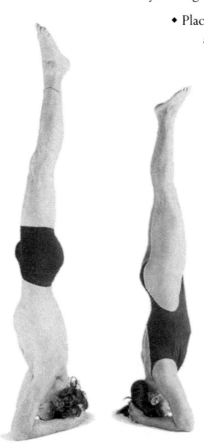

• Place the top of your head on the floor and clasp your hands around the back of your head (this "tripod" position is the foundation for the headstand).

• Without moving your head or arms, and with your feet on the floor, straighten your legs and push your hips up to an upside-down "V" position.

• Slowly walk your feet toward your face until your hips are aligned over your head.

• Holding the majority of your weight with your elbows and forearms, slowly bend your knees and lift your feet off the floor.

• Continue moving your feet toward the sky by straightening your knees and reaching up with your toes. Maintain length in your spine and neck as you breathe deeply.

• Maintaining the Headstand position, arch your back and slowly drop your legs toward your partner's legs. Once you make contact with your partner's feet or legs, keep this connection and press the insides of your legs together.

◆ Breathe and stabilize. Release your hands from the back of your head and place your palms on the floor beside your head (your forearms are about parallel).

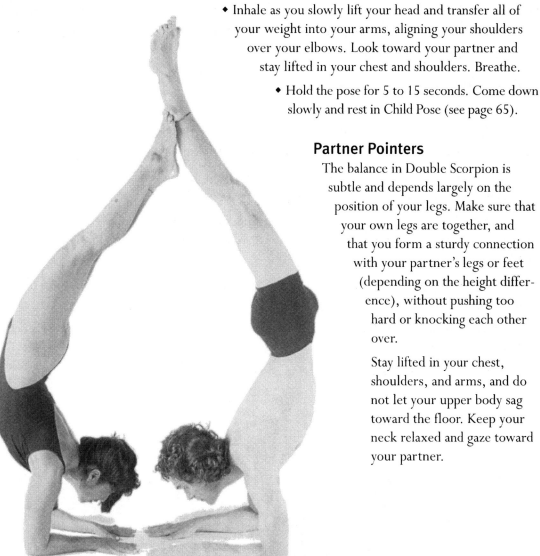

◆ Inhale as you slowly lift your head and transfer all of your weight into your arms, aligning your shoulders over your elbows. Look toward your partner and stay lifted in your chest and shoulders. Breathe.

◆ Hold the pose for 5 to 15 seconds. Come down slowly and rest in Child Pose (see page 65).

Partner Pointers

The balance in Double Scorpion is subtle and depends largely on the position of your legs. Make sure that your own legs are together, and that you form a sturdy connection with your partner's legs or feet (depending on the height difference), without pushing too hard or knocking each other over.

Stay lifted in your chest, shoulders, and arms, and do not let your upper body sag toward the floor. Keep your neck relaxed and gaze toward your partner.

CAUTIONS: Double Scorpion is not recommended for those with high blood pressure, a history of stroke, or acute spinal or neck injuries, or for women who are pregnant or menstruating.

Benefits

Builds upper-body strength ◆ Develops courage and willpower ◆ Improves mental clarity and concentration ◆ Gives the circulatory system a rest and potentially relieves varicose veins, hemorrhoids, and digestive disorders ◆ Helps balance the endocrine system

The Steeple

When you are feeling a bit dull or sluggish, practice The Steeple, a Partner Yoga hybrid of the Wheel Pose, *Chakrasana*. This invigorating back bend flushes the body with new energy and brings clarity to the mind.

TECHNIQUE

• Both partners, lie on your back, facing opposite directions, with your left hip about an inch from your partner's left hip.

• Place the palms of your hands under your shoulders, with your elbows pointing up.

• Keeping your knees and feet parallel (about hip-width apart), tuck your tailbone, push your feet into the floor, and begin to press the front of your hips toward the sky.

• Inhale, pressing your feet and hands firmly into the floor, and begin to arch your back while straightening your legs and arms. Exhale, stabilize your position, and root through your right foot.

• Inhale as you lift your left leg perpendicular to the floor. Bring the back of your calf or foot (depending on the height difference) together with your partner's calf or foot.

• Lengthen out through the lifted leg and reach up with your toes. Open through your shoulders and chest and breathe deeply.

• Hold the pose for 5 to 15 seconds. Come out slowly and rest in Corpse Pose.

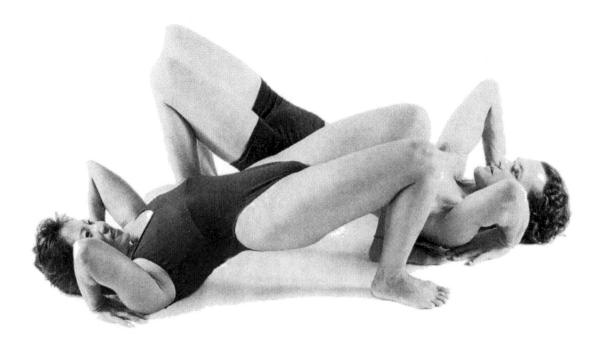

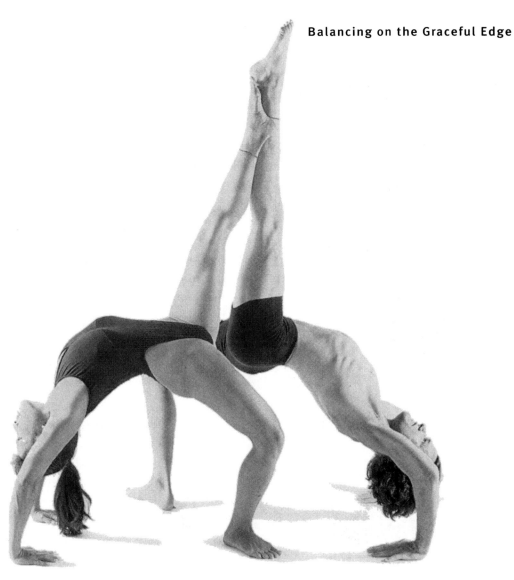

Partner Pointers

To avoid putting unnatural strain on the intervertebral discs, maintain length in your spine and keep your tailbone tucked throughout the entire work-up and completion of the pose.

As you lift your leg to meet your partner's leg, you may need to shift your position slightly so that your left hip moves in toward your partner. The pose is strongest when the lifted legs form a congruent line at the center of the pose.

NOTE: If you find that your base foot slips as you lift your opposing leg, place a sticky mat under your foot and root firmly through your heel.

CAUTIONS: The Steeple is not recommended for those with acute spinal or neck injuries. In addition, always warm up thoroughly before practicing a back bend.

Benefits

Revitalizes the body and mind ✦ Strengthens the arms and thighs ✦ Opens the hip flexors and shoulders ✦ Helps you break through self-imposed limitations

Front-Lift Work-Up to Lifted Cobra

The lifts are characterized by the location of the main fulcrum that supports the lift, the base partner's feet. In all of the front-lifting postures, the feet are placed on the hips of the partner being lifted. Front lifts are fun and easy to practice, and since the lifted partner is facing the ground, the possibility of falling seems less scary.

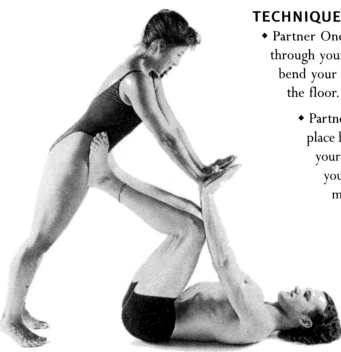

TECHNIQUE

♦ Partner One, lie on your back, rooting through your sacrum and lower back as you bend your knees and bring your feet off the floor.

♦ Partner Two, stand in front of One and place his feet on your hips. Begin to lean your weight forward into One's feet as you reach down with your hands to meet One's hands.

♦ Partner One, as Two leans her weight into your feet, allow your knees to bend and your thighs to move toward your chest. Lift your hands to meet Two's hands and breathe.

♦ This position is the foundation for the front lift.

♦ Partner Two, taking small steps toward your partner, continue to lean your weight into his feet and hands.

♦ Partner One, as your feet align over your hips, begin to straighten your knees and lift your partner off the ground. Once your legs are completely straight, keep your feet flat and your legs and arms perpendicular to the floor (in other words, keep your hands directly over your shoulders and your feet over your hips).

♦ Partner Two, press down with your hands into One's hands and straighten your arms. Slowly arch your back by lifting your head and chest. Straighten your legs and extend out through your toes. You are now in the Lifted Cobra.

♦ Both partners, breathe deeply and focus. Hold the pose for 10 to 30 seconds. Come down slowly, or move gracefully into another front lift posture such as The Falcon or the Hanging Forward Bend.

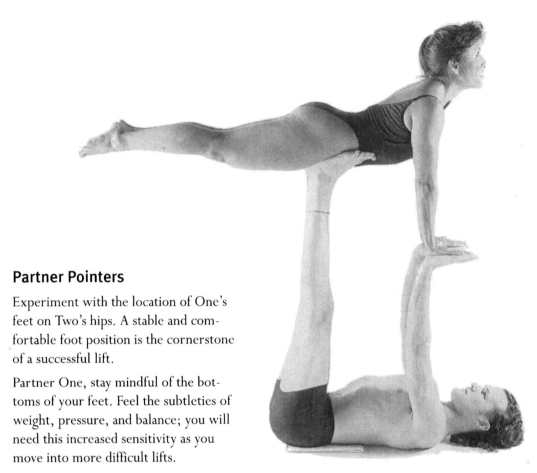

Partner Pointers

Experiment with the location of One's feet on Two's hips. A stable and comfortable foot position is the cornerstone of a successful lift.

Partner One, stay mindful of the bottoms of your feet. Feel the subtleties of weight, pressure, and balance; you will need this increased sensitivity as you move into more difficult lifts.

Partner Two, get in touch with any feelings you have about trust and surrender. Simply observe these feelings as they arise, and experience them fully with an underlying sense of detachment.

CAUTION: Lifts are advanced postures and can be dangerous if not performed correctly. Before attempting these postures, please read the specific cautions on page 132.

Benefits

Partner One

Strengthens the thighs and stretches the calves and hamstrings ◆ Brings new awareness to the sacrum and lower back, and promotes proper spinal alignment ◆ Massages the bottoms of the feet (Two's hipbones are a nice massage tool) ◆ Gives a much deserved break to veins in the legs and feet, relieving, and possibly preventing, varicose veins

Partner Two

Develops trust and courage ◆ Strengthens the back side of the body ◆ Induces feelings of lightness and freedom ◆ Heightens awareness of balance and interdependence

The Falcon

The Falcon is one of the most exhilarating of all the partner lifts. If you approach this pose with courage and unwavering focus, you will soar to new heights in body, mind, and spirit.

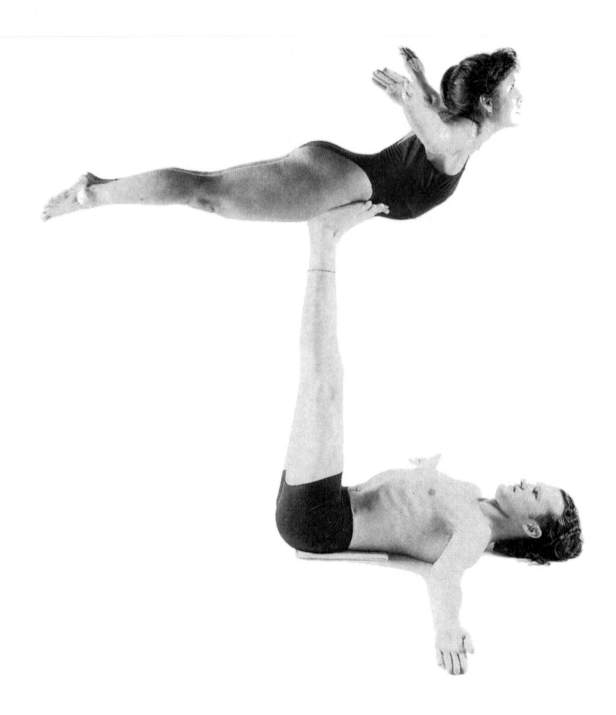

TECHNIQUE

• Begin by working into the Lifted Cobra. Breathe deeply as you get centered in the Lifted Cobra.

• Partner Two, inhale and slightly increase your upper-back arch, taking the weight off your hands (firmly engage the muscles of your back and buttocks). Holding your center perfectly still, slowly raise your arms out to your sides as you open through your chest and extend through your fingertips.

• Partner One, slowly lower your arms to the sides and rest them on the floor, palms up. Breathe deeply and use the power at your center to hold your feet, legs, and pelvis completely still.

• Both partners, stay focused and relaxed. Hold the pose as long as you wish.

• Come down slowly, or move directly into another forward lift position (we recommend Hanging Forward Bend; it is always wise to counter a back arch with a forward bend).

Partner Pointers

Partner One, bring increased awareness to the balls of your feet and your toes. Since you no longer have your arms to support Two's upper body, you must compensate by holding more weight with your toes (you may even need to position your feet slightly higher on Two's hips).

Partner Two, press firmly into One's feet with your hips and allow the rest of your body to lift up from this strong foundation. Keep your head lifted and your gaze just above the horizon.

CAUTION: Lifts are advanced postures and can be dangerous if not performed correctly. Before attempting these postures, please read the specific cautions on page 132.

Benefits

Partner One
> Strengthens the thighs and stretches the calves and hamstrings ◆ Brings new awareness to the sacrum and lower back, and promotes proper spinal alignment ◆ Massages the bottoms of the feet (Two's hipbones are a nice massage tool) ◆ Gives a much deserved break to veins in the legs and feet, relieving, and possibly preventing, varicose veins ◆ Deepens your concentration, integrating your body and mind in a single pointed focus

Partner Two
> Develops trust and courage ◆ Strengthens the back side of the body ◆ Induces feelings of lightness and freedom ◆ Heightens awareness of balance and interdependence ◆ Moves you past your perceived limitations ◆ Invokes sensations of flight and inner freedom

Hanging Forward Bend

The Hanging Forward Bend has produced more smiles and sighs of relief than any other Partner Yoga posture. This simple lift can relieve neck and back pain like a massage therapist and a chiropractor wrapped into one.

TECHNIQUE

◆ Begin in Lifted Cobra.

◆ Partner Two, exhale and slowly bend forward from your hips. Allow your legs to relax and your upper body and head to hang freely.

◆ Partner One, place your hands on Two's shoulders to help guide her torso smoothly into the forward bend. Once Two is all the way down, use your hands to rub and massage her neck, shoulders, and back (you can also gently pull down on the backs of her arms to create a light traction on her spine). Relax and breathe deeply.

◆ Hold the pose for as long as is comfortable. Come out slowly, or move directly to another front lift such as Hanging Straddle.

Partner Pointers

Partner One, make sure your feet stay over your hips and your legs remain perpendicular to the ground. With proper alignment, holding your partner's weight takes less strength and energy.

Partner Two, to fully experience this pose, you must completely let go. Imagine that you are surrendering to gravity; allow your entire body—as well as your thoughts, fears, and inhibitions—to melt into the pull of the Earth.

CAUTION: Lifts are advanced postures and can be dangerous if not performed correctly. Before attempting these postures, please read the cautions on page 132.

Benefits

Partner One
Strengthens the thighs and stretches the calves and hamstrings ◆ Brings new awareness to the sacrum and lower back, and promotes proper spinal alignment ◆ Massages the bottoms of the feet (Two's hipbones are a nice massage tool) ◆ Gives a much deserved break to veins in the legs and feet, relieving, and possibly preventing, varicose veins

Partner Two
Releases tension in the neck and shoulders ◆ Reverses normal downward (compressing) pressure on the spine ◆ Stimulates the abdominal organs ◆ Invokes deep feelings of surrender and acceptance

Hanging Straddle

This inverted pose uses the force of gravity to lengthen the spine and stretch the legs.

TECHNIQUE

♦ Begin in Hanging Forward Bend.

♦ Partner Two, slowly move your legs out to the side and reach your hands toward your feet. Hold your big toe with your thumb and forefinger. Relax your shoulders and neck, and surrender to gravity. As you breathe, feel your back and shoulders widening and the muscles in your legs becoming more elastic.

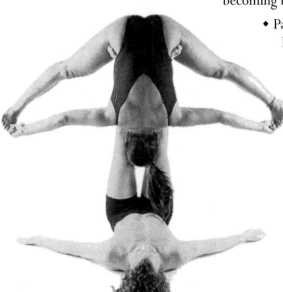

♦ Partner One, maintain length in your legs and hold steady as you relax your arms out to the sides and breathe deeply.

♦ Hold the pose for as long as you wish.

Partner Pointers

Partner One, to hold a strong foundation, you must keep your knees straight and your legs perpendicular to the floor.

Partner Two, focus on breathing into your arms, legs, and spine. Feel as if your entire body is lengthening and becoming more elastic.

CAUTION: Lifts are advanced postures and can be dangerous if not performed correctly. Before attempting these postures, please read the specific cautions on page 132.

Benefits

Partner One

Strengthens the thighs and stretches the calves and hamstrings ♦ Brings new awareness to the sacrum and lower back, and promotes proper spinal alignment ♦ Massages the bottoms of the feet (Two's hipbones are a nice massage tool) ♦ Gives a much deserved break to veins in the legs and feet, relieving, and possibly preventing, varicose veins

Partner Two

Releases tension in the neck and shoulders ♦ Reverses normal downward (compressing) pressure on the spine ♦ Stimulates the abdominal organs ♦ Invokes deep feelings of surrender and acceptance ♦ Stretches the hamstrings and inner thighs ♦ Opens the chest and shoulders, and deepens your breathing

Back-Lift Work-Up to Lifted Back Bend

In the back-lift postures, the main point of contact is the base partner's feet on the lifted partner's sacrum. Yogis believe there is a potent spiritual energy—brilliant as a million suns—called *kundalini shakti* that lies dormant at the base of the spine near the sacrum. Through heightened awareness of the subtleties of the spine and sacrum, one begins the process of awakening the *kundalini shakti*.

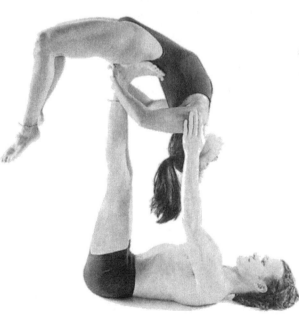

TECHNIQUE

◆ Partner One, lie on your back, lengthen your spine, and root your sacrum and lower back into the floor. Bend your knees toward your chest and bring your feet off the floor.

◆ Partner Two, place One's feet on your sacrum, with his toes on the middle part of your lower back. Bend your knees and begin to lean your weight back into One's feet in a sitting motion. Support yourself with your hands on One's shins (use your hands to hold a firm connection to One's feet).

◆ Partner One, as Two leans her weight into your feet, allow your thighs to move further toward your chest. Lift your hands to Two's elbows for added support. This position is the foundation for all the back lift postures.

◆ Partner Two, take a few small steps back toward One, progressively leaning more of your weight onto One's feet.

◆ Partner One, as your feet align over your hips, slowly begin to straighten your knees and lift Two off the floor. Once your legs are straight, make sure your sacrum is flat on the floor and your legs are perpendicular to the floor. Continue supporting Two through shoulder contact.

◆ Partner Two, as you feel comfortable and stable, let go of One's shins and stretch your arms overhead.

◆ Partner One, relax your arms to the floor with the palms of your hands up.

◆ Both partners, breathe deeply and focus. Hold the pose for as long as you like.

◆ Come down slowly, or move directly to the Lifted Bow.

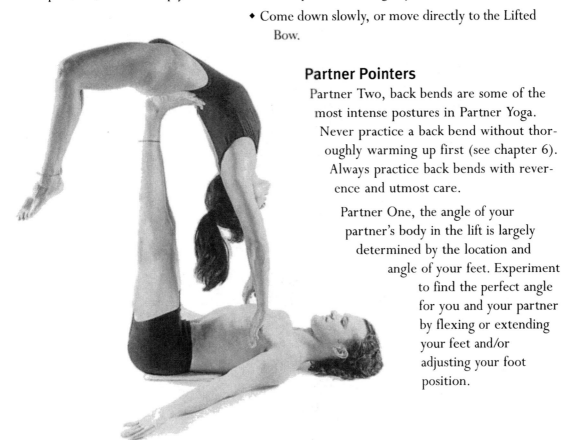

Partner Pointers

Partner Two, back bends are some of the most intense postures in Partner Yoga. Never practice a back bend without thoroughly warming up first (see chapter 6). Always practice back bends with reverence and utmost care.

Partner One, the angle of your partner's body in the lift is largely determined by the location and angle of your feet. Experiment to find the perfect angle for you and your partner by flexing or extending your feet and/or adjusting your foot position.

CAUTIONS: Lifts are advanced postures and can be dangerous if not performed correctly. Before attempting these postures, please read the specific cautions on page 132. In addition, always warm up thoroughly before practicing a back bend.

Benefits

Partner One

Strengthens the thighs and stretches the calves and hamstrings ◆ Brings increased awareness to the sacrum and lower back, and promotes proper spinal alignment ◆ Heightens awareness of balance and interdependence

Partner Two

Increases circulation in the abdomen and lungs ◆ Limbers the iliopsoas muscles (hip flexors) and spine ◆ Stimulates the kidneys and adrenal glands ◆ Releases fear and other stuck emotions

Lifted Bow

The Lifted Bow is a variation of *Danurasana*, the Bow Pose. This invigorating lift augments the benefits of the Lifted Back Bend by opening the shoulders and chest and stimulating the heart.

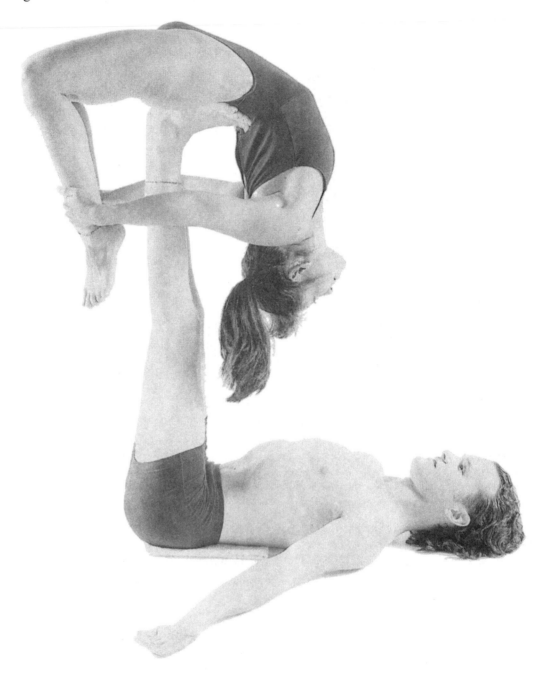

TECHNIQUE

◆ Begin in Lifted Back Bend.

◆ Partner Two, inhale and lengthen your spine as you slowly bend your knees and reach your hands to your ankles or shins. Open through your chest, stay aware of your balance, and breathe deeply.

◆ Partner One, hold steady and keep your breathing smooth and consistent and your legs perpendicular to the ground.

Partner Pointers

Partner Two, never practice a back bend without thoroughly warming up first (see chapter 6). Always practice back bends with reverence and utmost care.

Partner Two, as you reach for your ankles, do not allow your upper back (between your shoulder blades) to close off. Think of this area as the "back door of the heart," and keep this area open by filling it with breath.

Partner One, as Two reaches for her ankles, you may need to adjust the tilt of your feet to maintain the most effective balance.

Partner Two, to avoid strain on your lower back, engage your buttocks, tuck your tailbone, and stay lengthened throughout your entire spine.

Partrer Two, if you begin to fall, remember to release your ankles and roll gently to the ground. Partner One, be sure to release any hold you have on Partner Two, and simply provide general support in assisting Partner Two to the ground, without gripping or holding onto her.

CAUTIONS: Lifts are advanced postures and can be dangerous if not performed correctly. Before attempting these postures, please read the specific cautions on page 132. Always warm up thoroughly before practicing a back bend. If reaching your hands to your ankles makes the back bend too intense, simply return to Lifted Back Bend. Be patient with your spine and never force anything; with time the flexibility will come.

Benefits

Partner One

Strengthens the thighs and stretches the calves and hamstrings ◆ Brings increased awareness to the sacrum and lower back, and promotes proper spinal alignment ◆ Heightens awareness of balance and interdependence

Partner Two

Increases circulation in the abdomen and lungs ◆ Limbers the iliopsoas muscles (hip flexors) and spine ◆ Stimulates the kidneys and adrenal glands ◆ Releases fear and other stuck emotions ◆ Opens the heart and throat, and produces feelings of expansiveness ◆ Increases flexibility in the shoulders and chest

Upper-Back Lift Work-Up to Lifted Upper-Back Arch

The upper-back lifts are some of the most interesting to practice. The weight distribution and nuances of balance are unlike any of the other Partner Yoga lifts. As you practice these lifts, listen to your intuition and have fun.

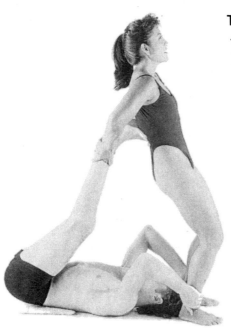

TECHNIQUE

◆ Partner One, lie on your back and align your spine and hips. Bend your knees and lift your legs so that your feet rest above your face (your sacrum will lift off the ground slightly).

◆ Partner Two, stand with your feet just in front of One's head and place his feet in the middle of your upper back. With your hands on One's ankles, bend your knees and begin to lean your weight back into One's feet.

◆ Partner One, reach your hands to Two's ankles with your elbows facing up. This is the foundation for the upper-back lifts.

◆ Partner One, as Two leans her weight into your feet, allow your sacrum to roll back toward the ground. As your feet start to align over your hips, lift Two's feet off the ground and straighten your arms overhead.

◆ Both partners, breathe and stabilize.

◆ Partner Two, inhale as you extend your arms overhead, palms together, and lengthen your entire body from head to toe. Exhale and settle into a graceful back bend.

◆ Partner One, hold steady and breathe deep.

◆ Hold the pose for as long as you like. Come down slowly, or move directly into Lifted Camel.

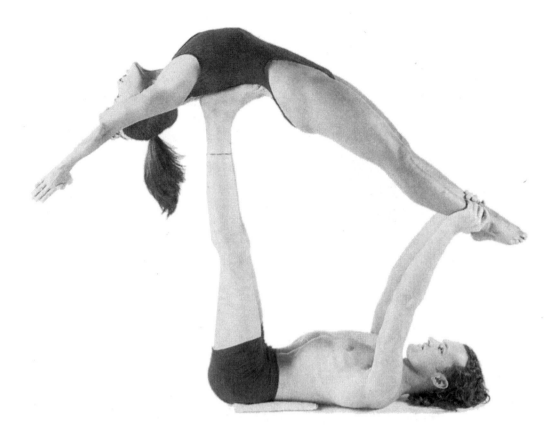

Partner Pointers

Both partners, the subtleties of this lift—such as foot position and leg angles—will be different for everyone. Keep the channels of communication open and figure out what works best for you.

CAUTION: Lifts are advanced postures and can be dangerous if not performed correctly. Before attempting these postures, please read the specific cautions on page 132.

Benefits

Partner One

Strengthens the thighs, hips, and abdominal muscles ◆ Gives a much deserved break to veins in the legs and feet, relieving, and possibly preventing, varicose veins ◆ Builds upper-body strength (particularly the triceps and pectoral muscles) ◆ Heightens awareness of balance and weight distribution

Partner Two

Increases flexibility in the mid- and upper back (many people have limited mobility in the upper thoracic spine) ◆ Opens the chest, ribs, and shoulders, making deep breathing easier ◆ Produces feelings of lightness and grace

Lifted Camel

The Lifted Camel is a creative variation of the traditional Camel Pose, *Ustrasana*. This invigorating pose does wonders for opening and expanding the heart.

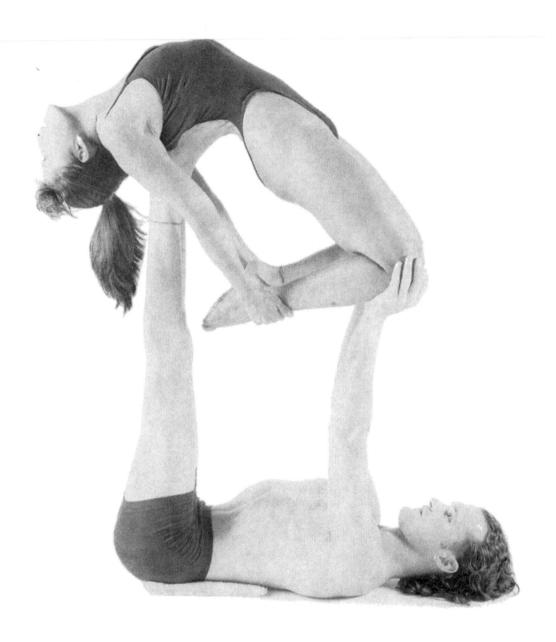

TECHNIQUE

• Begin in Lifted Upper-Back Arch.

• Partner One, holding Two's right ankle steady in your left hand, slowly shift the position of your right hand up to Two's knee by sliding your hand up her shin. Immediately begin to shift your left hand into the same position, holding Two's right knee. As you make this transition, push slightly with your toes; this will transfer more of Two's weight into your legs and lighten the load on your arms.

• Partner One, once you have both of Two's knees in your palms, straighten your arms and relax your shoulders.

• Partner Two, as your knees bend, reach your hands down to your ankles and open through your chest and shoulders. Maintain a long spine and allow your head to gently drop back, opening your throat toward the sky. Breathe smooth and consistent.

• Hold the pose for as long as you like. Come down slowly and rest in Child Pose.

Partner Pointers

Moving from the Lifted Upper-Back Arch to the Camel can be kind of tricky. Use the techniques we have explained, and also follow your creative intuition.

Partner One, you may have to experiment to find the best foot position to support Two's back. Move consciously and communicate with each other.

As always, be patient with yourself and your partner, and, most important, enjoy the process.

CAUTIONS: Lifts are advanced postures and can be dangerous if not performed correctly. Before attempting these postures, please read the specific cautions on page 132. In addition, always warm up thoroughly before practicing a back bend.

Benefits

Partner One
> Strengthens the thighs, hips, and abdominal muscles ◆ Gives a much deserved break to veins in the legs and feet, relieving, and possibly preventing, varicose veins ◆ Builds upper-body strength (particularly the triceps and pectoral muscles) ◆ Heightens awareness of balance and weight distribution

Partner Two
> Increases flexibility in the upper back and neck ◆ Stretches the iliopsoas muscles (hip flexors) and quadriceps (thigh muscles) ◆ Opens the shoulders, chest, and ribs ◆ Awakens enthusiasm and zest for life

Seated-Lift Work-Up to Lifted Chair

Okay, we'll admit, the Lifted Chair is a pretty silly pose. We originally used this position as an intermediate pose before working into Lifted Lotus. Later, we realized the Lifted Chair is a fun pose to practice on its own—especially on those shaky days when Lifted Lotus seems way too scary.

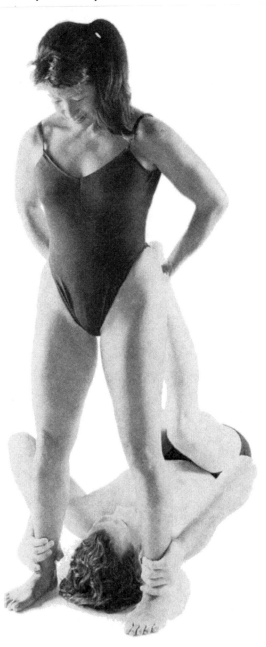

TECHNIQUE

• Partner One, lie on your back and align your spine and hips.

• Partner One, bend your knees and lift your legs so that your feet rest above your face (your sacrum will lift off the ground slightly).

• Partner Two, stand with your feet just in front of One's head and position the arches of his feet directly under your sitz bones.

• Partner Two, with your hands on One's ankles, bend your knees and begin to lean your weight into One's feet as if sitting in a chair.

• Partner One, reach your hands to Two's ankles with your elbows facing up. This is the foundation for the seated lifts.

• Partner One, as Two leans her weight into your feet, allow your sacrum to roll back toward the ground. As your feet start to align over your hips, lift Two's feet off the ground and straighten your legs.

• Partner One, as you steady the pose, bring the palms of your hands under Two's feet and position your arms parallel to your legs.

• Partner Two, root your sitz bones into One's feet and sit with your spine erect and your shoulders relaxed.

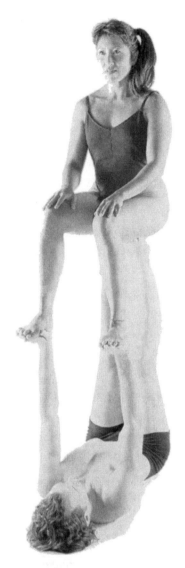

• Both partners, steady your breathing and still your mind.

• Hold the Lifted Chair for as long as you like. Come down slowly, or move directly into Lifted Lotus.

Partner Pointers

Partner One, as you lift Partner Two, adjust your foot position as needed to find the most stable location on Partner Two's sitz bones.

Partner One, create a sturdy base with your hands for Two's feet to rest upon. Keep your arms active and your shoulders relaxed.

Partner Two, avoid making large or quick movements. Keep your upper body erect and hold steady at your center. It may help your balance to hold a soft gaze at the horizon.

Both partners, breathe deeply and stay calm.

In the event that Partner Two starts to fall, Partner One must let go of her feet so she can safely land with her feet on the ground.

Partner Two, if you fall, make sure you widen your feet enough to clear One's body as you land.

CAUTION: Lifts are advanced postures and can be dangerous if not performed correctly. Before attempting these postures, please read the specific cautions on page 132.

Benefits

Partner One
> Strengthens the thighs, hips, and abdominal muscles ◆ Gives a much deserved break to veins in the legs and feet, relieving, and possibly preventing, varicose veins ◆ Builds upper-body strength (particularly the triceps and pectoral muscles) ◆ Heightens awareness of balance and weight distribution

Partner Two
> Improves awareness of posture ◆ Reminds you to be playful, and usually produces a good laugh or two ◆ Provides a place to sit while you contemplate practicing the Lifted Lotus

Lifted Lotus

The Lifted Lotus is undoubtedly the most challenging partner posture in this book. This pose is recommended only for advanced yogis or those who can successfully perform all of the other partner lifts.

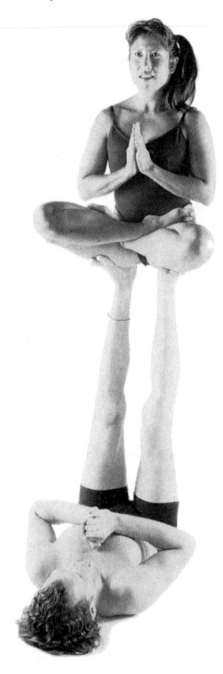

TECHNIQUE

◆ Start in Lifted Chair.

◆ Both partners, slow your breathing, calm your mind, and bring your entire being into a single pointed focus (the intense state of concentration yogis refer to as *dharana*).

◆ Partner Two, root your sitz bones firmly into One's feet by allowing your breath to drop down into your lower belly.

◆ Partner Two, slowly lift one leg and, using your hands, guide your foot to the top of your thigh in half lotus. Holding your center perfectly still, lift your other leg and place your foot on the opposite thigh.

◆ Partner Two, gaze at the horizon and bring your palms together in front of your heart. Breathe.

◆ Partner One, bring your palms together at your heart, breathe, and hold perfectly still.

◆ Hold the pose for as long as you feel comfortable and focused.

VARIATION: Ancient yoga texts describe a lotus flower with 1,000 luminous petals that resides at the crown of the head. The unfolding of this lotus represents the attainment of spiritual enlightenment. In this variation of Lifted Lotus, hold your hands above the crown of your head as a way of honoring the great lotus (*padma*) within each of us.

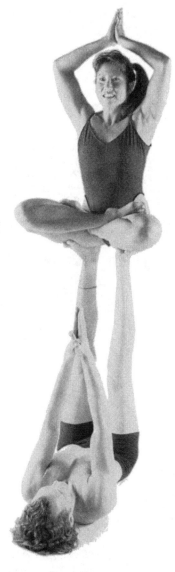

Partner Pointers

The Lotus Pose, *Padmasana*, is one of the most sacred poses in yoga. Always approach this partner lift with reverence and humility.

As you practice the Lifted Lotus, confront your challenges—be they mental or physical—with what we call mindful courage (see chapter 12). In other words, be totally present and truthful with yourself, your partner, and the challenges you face together.

Smile within.

NOTE: When you're first learning the Lifted Lotus, it is a good idea to have a third person present to serve as a spotter. The spotter can support the lifted partner if she needs to adjust her position and/or help prevent a dangerous fall.

CAUTION: Lifts are advanced postures and can be dangerous if not performed correctly. Before attempting these postures, please read the specific cautions on page 132.

Benefits

Partner One

Strengthens the thighs, hips, and abdominal muscles ◆ Gives a much deserved break to veins in the legs and feet, relieving, and possibly preventing, varicose veins ◆ Heightens awareness of balance and weight distribution ◆ Brings the mind into a single pointed focus (Advanced yogis, this is the perfect opportunity to practice the sixth limb of yoga, *dharana*.) ◆ Intensely heightens awareness of the feet, legs, and hips

Partner Two

Gives an opportunity to closely examine fear and trust

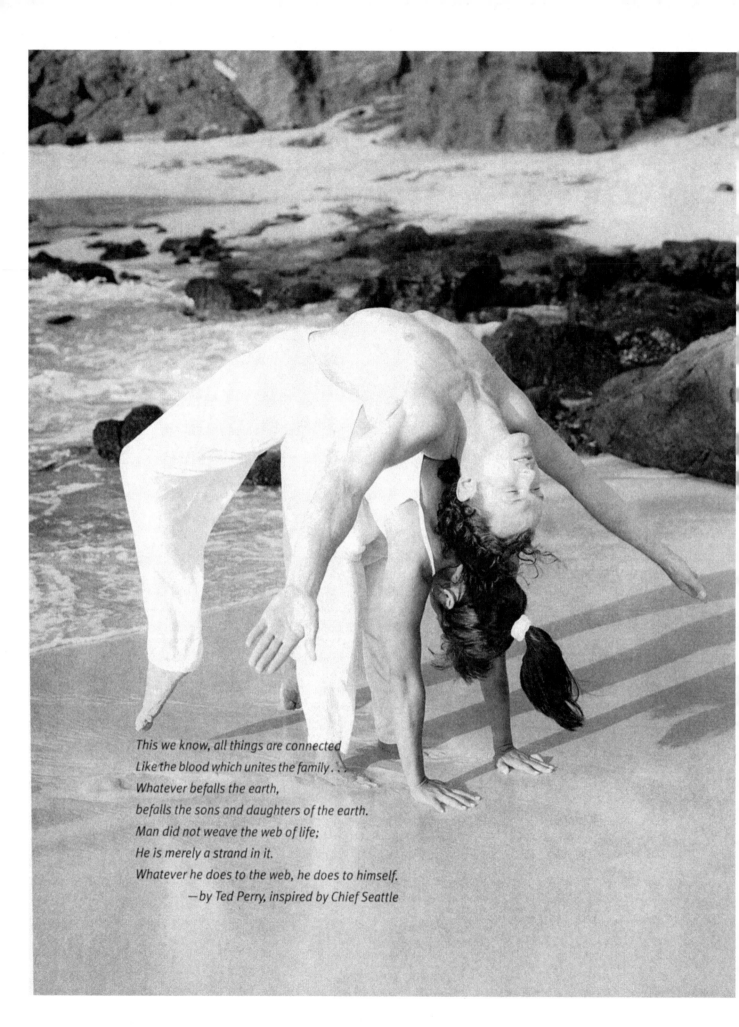

This we know, all things are connected
Like the blood which unites the family . . .
Whatever befalls the earth,
befalls the sons and daughters of the earth.
Man did not weave the web of life;
He is merely a strand in it.
Whatever he does to the web, he does to himself.
—by Ted Perry, inspired by Chief Seattle

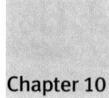

Chapter 10

Partner Flows

"My yoga practice became a flowing uncensored music of the soul that felt more like a prayer than a practice of postures."

—Yogi Amrit Desai, author of *Meditation in Motion*

What does it mean to flow? A river moving downstream is flowing. Often there are rocks or other obstructions in its way, yet it still flows. Water moves around the rocks or fallen branches and somehow continues on its way. Whether it is a quiet day or there is a raging storm, there is still the continuous flow of water. The movement, however slight, does not ever stop.

So it is with our lives. From the moment we take our first breaths, we are in a continuous flow. We may attempt to compartmentalize our lives into different events: work, vacation, play, rest. Yet these events are all part of the same flow of life. They are truly interdependent and interconnected. For example, many people have jobs where they are stressed and overworked. Everyday they look forward to getting off work or to an approaching vacation where they will finally be able to relax. When it is time to go home or on vacation, they put work behind them and move on to this perceived "next event." They keep these events separate, sighing with deep relief as work is done and "after-work" begins.

The truth is that what happens at work significantly affects what happens at home. If we are stressed at work, we bring that stress, in one way or another, into whatever else we do. It might make us withdraw, yell at our partners, or take it out on the kids. Similarly, if we do not get our needs met at home—rest, play, support, affection—our performance and attitude at work are affected. All things are interdependent.

In Partner Yoga flows, we practice poses in a sequence to increase our awareness of how one thing connects to the next. The poses are practiced in a continuous stream of movement in constant contact with your partner. Rest is integrated into each pose, so there is no rest between postures. During a flow, every breath and movement is yoga. Once you begin to feel the connection between movements, you become more aware of the connection among all aspects of life.

What follows are three Partner Yoga flows: The Quick Flow, The Power Flow, and The Relax Flow. Each flow offers a unique experience. If you have limited time, practice the Quick Flow. If you are in need of an invigorating workout, give the Power Flow a go. The Relax Flow is a perfect way to unwind after a long day.

When starting a Partner Yoga flow or, for that matter, any Partner Yoga session, remember the importance of bringing awareness to the breath first. Breathe into your chest, back, and abdomen. Feel the breath move into every cell. Let your mind release scattered thoughts, and allow yourself to be fully present. General guidelines are given for how long to hold each pose. As always, do what feels best for you. If you feel the need to hold poses longer or move through them quicker, follow your inner rhythm.

The Quick Flow

This sequence was born out of the need to stretch tight legs and sore butts after sitting on long airplane or car rides. When we found ourselves needing to stretch in dirty airports or rest stops, sitting postures just didn't cut it. We needed effective standing postures that could be done quickly. So we created this flow, nicknamed "Flow on the Go" because it takes only about 10 minutes and can be done just about anywhere.

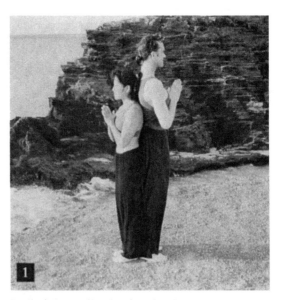

Begin by standing back to back in Twin Peaks (see page 66) with your hands together at your heart. Breathe and become aware of the connection between you and your partner. Remember to breathe deeply throughout the entire flow.

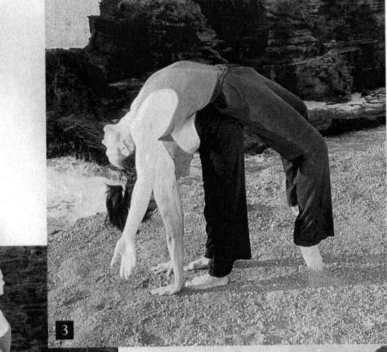

3

Partner Two, move into the forward bend as you exhale and lift Partner One over your back. Hold for a few breaths.

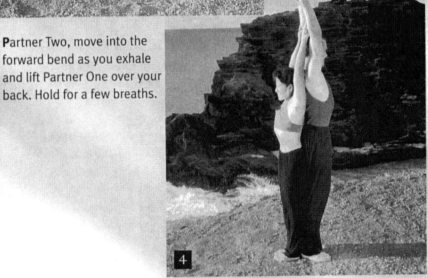

2

Reach behind and link elbows with your partner, preparing for The Backpack (see page 102).

4

Return to Twin Peaks, stretch your arms overhead, and lengthen your spine (see page 66).
Link arms with your partner once again. Partner One, lift Partner Two over your back (not shown here). Hold for a few breaths.
Once again return to Twin Peaks with your arms extended up.

(continued)

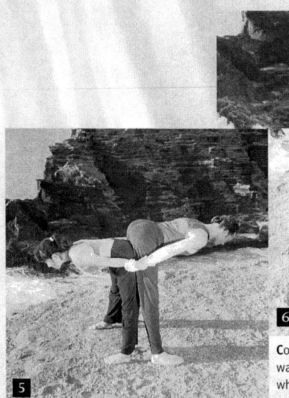

5

Widen your stance until your feet are about 3 feet apart. Link hands, exhale, and bend forward from your hips. Bend until your backs are parallel to the ground, with your buttocks and backs of thighs pressing together.

6

Continue to bend all the way toward the ground while maintaining length in your spine. Lengthen through the backs of your legs. Adjust your hand position and settle into Standing Straddle (see page 76). Hold for a few breaths.

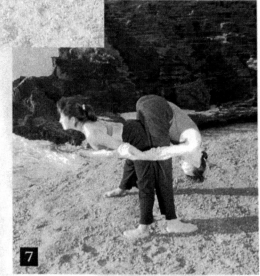

7

Partner Two, inhale, look up, and lift your torso parallel to the ground. This will bring Partner One into a deeper hamstring stretch while strengthening your lower and mid-back muscles. This movement is an adaptation of the technique shown in The Pump (see page 74). Both partners alternate performing this pumping action.

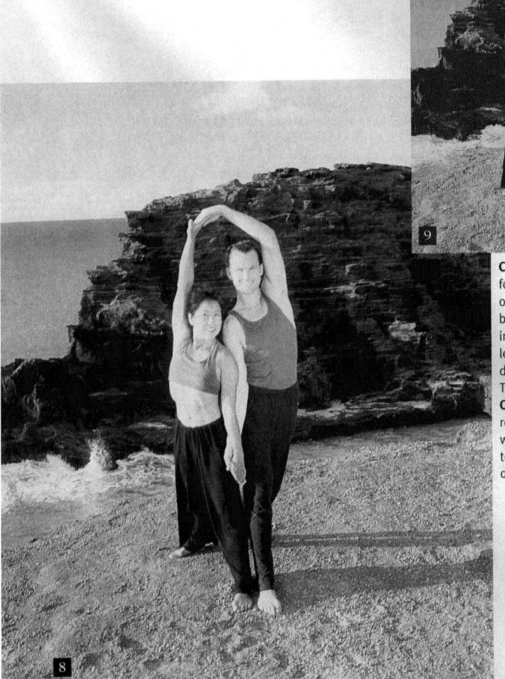

9

8

Complete the turn by extending forward with the arm that is overhead. Bring the other arm behind you and press your hip in toward your partner. Inhale, lengthen your spine, and move deeper into the Standing Double Twist (see page 104).

Come out of the twist slowly and return standing back to back with your arms outstretched to your sides. Repeat on the opposite side.

(continued)

Return to standing back to back with your arms outstretched to your sides. Partner One, turn toward your right and Partner Two, turn toward your left, lowering the arm that is in the direction of the turn, and raising the other arm overhead.

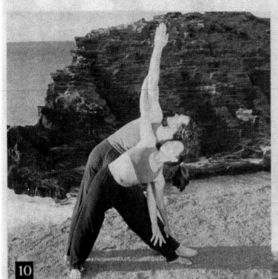

Once again, return to standing back to back with your arms outstretched to your sides and begin moving into Double Triangle (see page 106). Keeping your buttocks and backs pressed together, exhale and begin bending to the side. Cross arms with your partner so your lower arm is on your partner's shin or ankle and your upper arm is reaching to the sky. Gaze upward and breathe.

10

11

Return standing upright with out-stretched arms. Both partners, bend your knee and lunge into Double Warrior B (see page 77). Make sure your bent knee stays over your ankle and your shinbone is perpendicular to the ground. **R**elax your shoulders and look toward your outstretched arm on the side of your bent knee. Hold for a few breaths. Repeat Double Triangle and Double Warrior B on the other side (not shown here).

12

Turn and stand side by side, facing the same direction. Reach your arm around your partner's back.

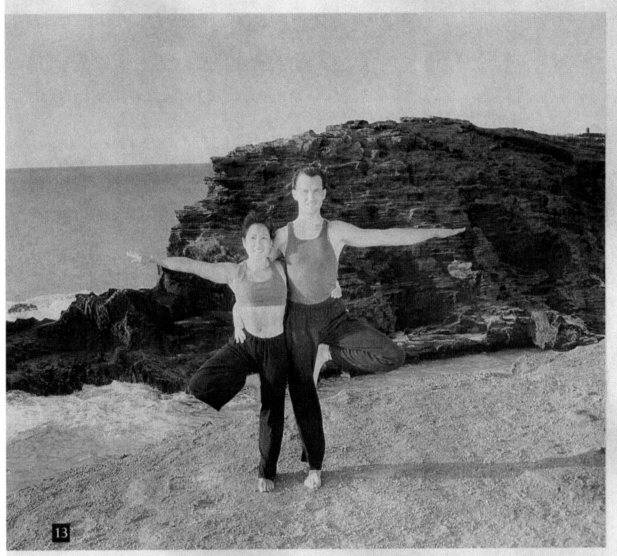

13

Lift your outside foot to the inner thigh of your standing leg. Extend your outside arm out to the side in Double Tree (see page 133). Breathe and balance. Repeat on the opposite side.

(continued)

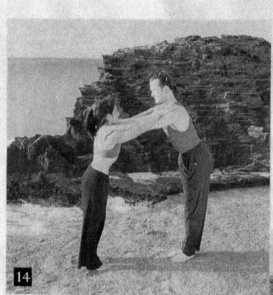

14

Still in contact with your partner, turn to face each other. Reach your hands to each other's shoulders in preparation for The Table (see page 68).

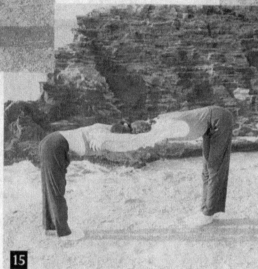

16

Begin to walk forward slowly while lifting your upper body. Continue holding your partner's hands, wrists, or forearms, and step forward until your feet are about 1 to 2 feet apart. Inhale, lengthen your spine, and begin to lean back, pressing your hips forward slightly.

15

Adjust your arm and hand position as you exhale, slowly bending forward and stepping back as you bring the tops of your heads together. As your upper bodies come parallel to the ground, lengthen through your spine and the backs of your legs. Hold for a few breaths.

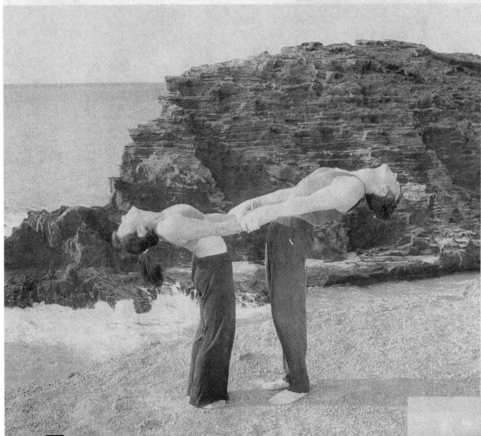

17

Relax and move slowly back into the full Fountain Pose (see page 98). Adjust your hand position as needed to create the most stable counterbalance position. Hold for a few breaths.

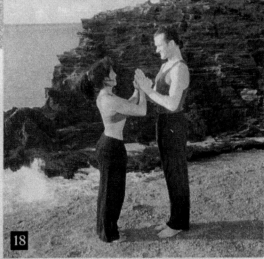

18

To finish the flow, face your partner and bring your hands together in front of your heart. Take a deep breath and, in your own way, extend a gesture of honor and appreciation to your partner.

The Power Flow

The second flow is called the Power Flow. Poses in this flow are generally held for 10 to 15 seconds longer than in the Quick Flow, without resting or stopping between the poses. The Power Flow is a total-being workout. The sequence includes postures that require strength, stamina, flexibility, trust, surrender, and balance. This flow activates your internal organs and all parts of your body from the tips of your toes to the top of your head.

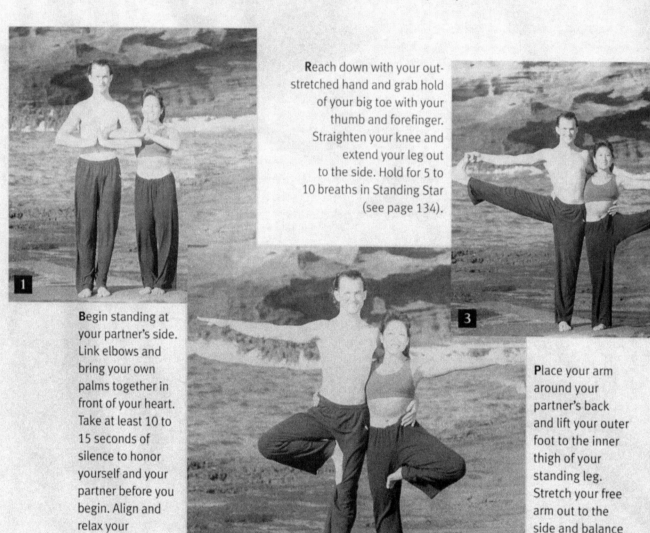

Reach down with your outstretched hand and grab hold of your big toe with your thumb and forefinger. Straighten your knee and extend your leg out to the side. Hold for 5 to 10 breaths in Standing Star (see page 134).

Begin standing at your partner's side. Link elbows and bring your own palms together in front of your heart. Take at least 10 to 15 seconds of silence to honor yourself and your partner before you begin. Align and relax your body/mind and breathe deeply into your back, chest, and abdomen.

Place your arm around your partner's back and lift your outer foot to the inner thigh of your standing leg. Stretch your free arm out to the side and balance in Double Tree pose (see page 133). Hold for 10 or more breaths.

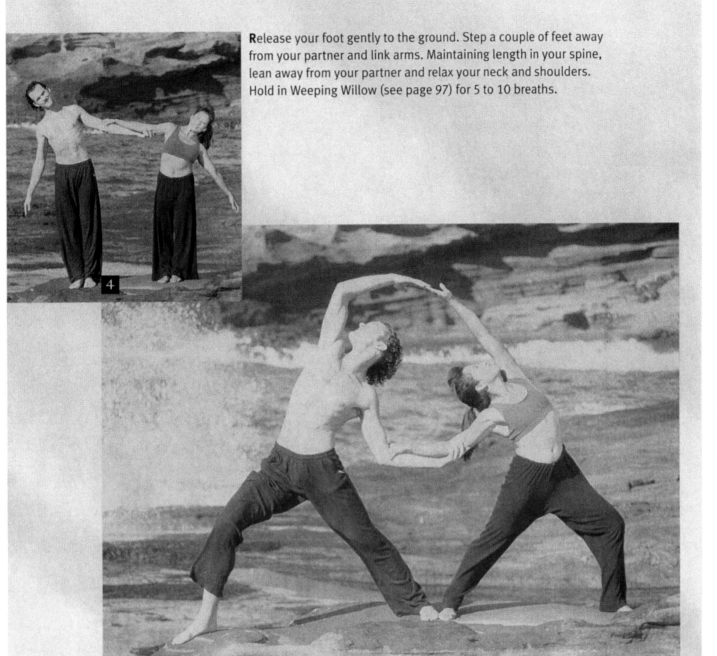

Release your foot gently to the ground. Step a couple of feet away from your partner and link arms. Maintaining length in your spine, lean away from your partner and relax your neck and shoulders. Hold in Weeping Willow (see page 97) for 5 to 10 breaths.

To stretch the other side of your body, move into The Gateway (see page 100). Step in toward your partner so that your inside foot presses against your partner's foot, and step out into a lunge with your other foot. Your inside foot will be facing straight ahead. Point your outer foot out toward the side you lunged to. Make sure your knee doesn't go beyond your ankle as you lunge. Reach up with your outside hand to meet your partner's hand. Exhale, look up, and hold for 5 to 10 breaths.

(continued)

Return to your upright
position. Repeat the last four
postures on the opposite side.

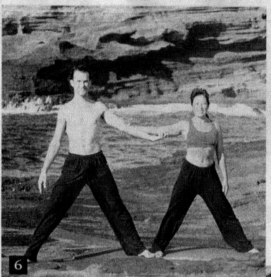

Exhale and take a large step out to
the side, both partners stepping in
the same direction. Keep your back
in contact with your partner, and
place your hand on the ground next
to the foot you just lunged with.

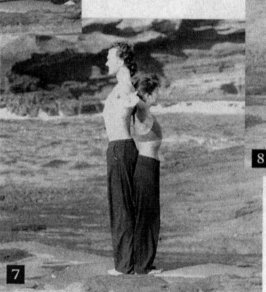

Turn back to back, maintaining arm contact.
Bring your feet together and stretch both your
arms out to the sides. Lengthen out through
your spine, relax, and breathe deeply.

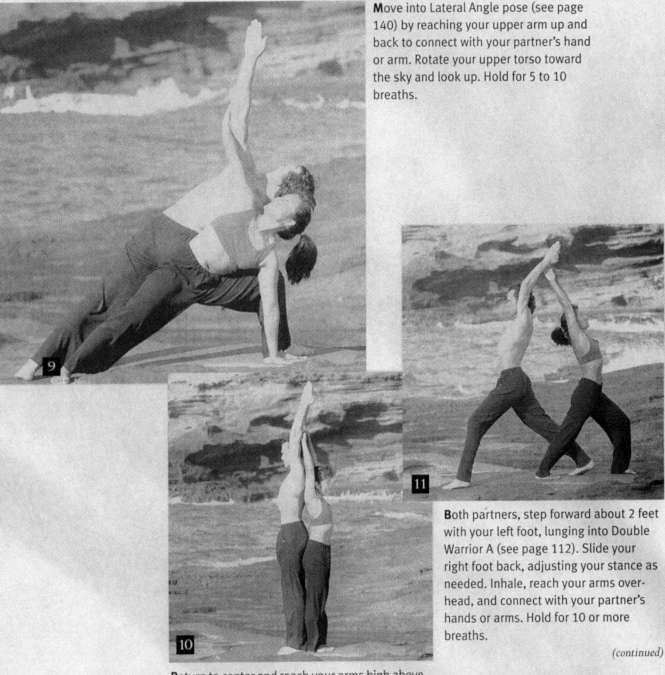

Move into Lateral Angle pose (see page 140) by reaching your upper arm up and back to connect with your partner's hand or arm. Rotate your upper torso toward the sky and look up. Hold for 5 to 10 breaths.

Both partners, step forward about 2 feet with your left foot, lunging into Double Warrior A (see page 112). Slide your right foot back, adjusting your stance as needed. Inhale, reach your arms overhead, and connect with your partner's hands or arms. Hold for 10 or more breaths.

(continued)

Return to center and reach your arms high above your head in Twin Peaks pose (see page 66). Lunge with your opposite foot and move into Lateral Angle pose on the other side. Return once again to Twin Peaks, reaching your arms overhead as you inhale. Relax your shoulders as you exhale.

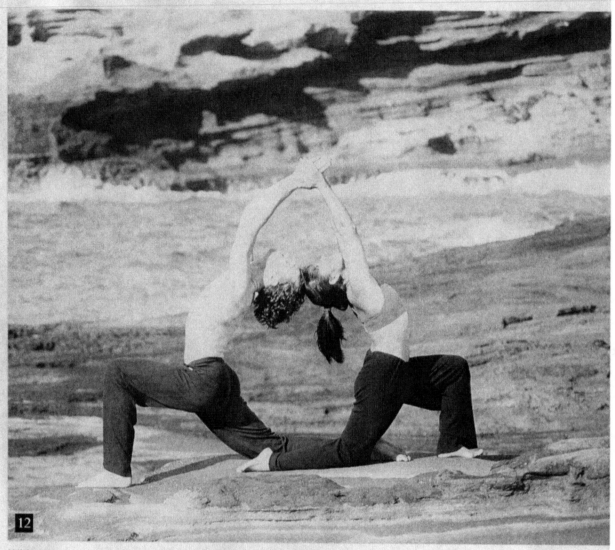

12

Widen your stance and sink down until your left thigh is parallel to the ground and your right knee and shin are resting on the ground. Use each other for support as you lower down. Inhale, tuck your tailbone, and lift your heart. Exhale, arch back, and touch the tops of your heads in The Porthole (see page 110). Hold for five or more breaths.

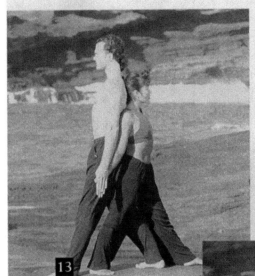

Return to center, standing with your hands linked and arms down to your sides. Leave your right leg behind you and your left leg in front of you, about 2 to 3 feet apart. Inhale and lengthen your spine.

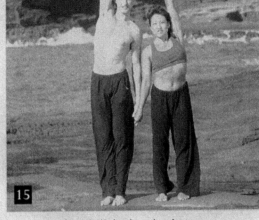

Exhale and bend forward at your hips, maintaining arm-to-arm contact as you bring your upper body over your front leg. Think of reaching toward the ground with the top of your head in The Umbrella pose (see page 78). Hold for 5 to 10 breaths. Return to center and step forward with your right leg, repeating the last four poses on the other side.

Keep your hands linked and spin to the side.

(continued)

Step in as you lift your upper body and link wrists with your partner. Bend your knees and lower into a chair position. Your knees are directly over your ankles and your thighs are parallel to the ground. Hold for 3 to 5 breaths (longer if you like).

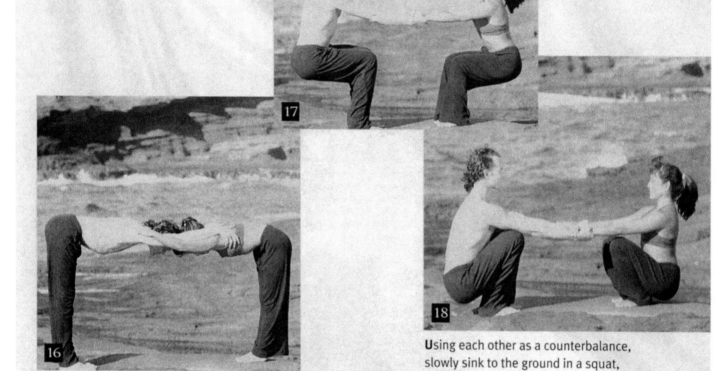

Continue your spin until you are standing face to face with your partner. Move your hands to your partner's shoulders as you take a few steps back. **E**xhale and bend forward at your hips until your back is parallel to the ground in The Table pose (see page 68). Relax and hold for 10 or more breaths.

Using each other as a counterbalance, slowly sink to the ground in a squat, being mindful of your knees.

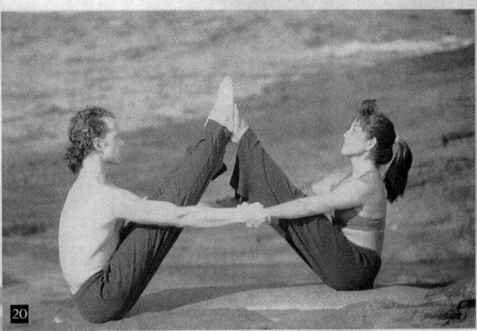

When you feel balanced, lift your other foot up so both legs are pointing toward the sky at about 45 degrees, and the bottoms of your feet are touching. Keep your arms parallel to the ground. Inhale, lift your chest, and lengthen your spine. Hold for 5 to 10 breaths in Double Boat (see page 116).

(continued)

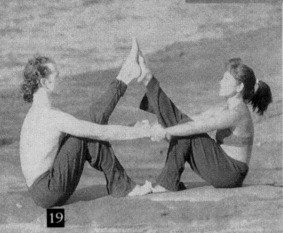

Sit gently on the ground while still holding each other's wrists. Both of your knees are bent and your toes are touching. Inhale and lengthen your spine as you lift one leg up, maintaining sole-to-sole contact with your partner's foot.

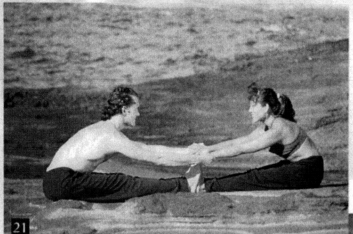

With your wrists still linked, lower your legs one by one and straighten them on the ground. Continue pressing your feet into your partner's feet as you bend slowly forward from your hips. Hold for 10 or more breaths in Double Seated Forward Bend (see page 79).

Slowly straighten your legs out to the side into Double Straddle (see page 118), keeping your knees and toes facing up. Breathe and hold the pose for 10 or more breaths.

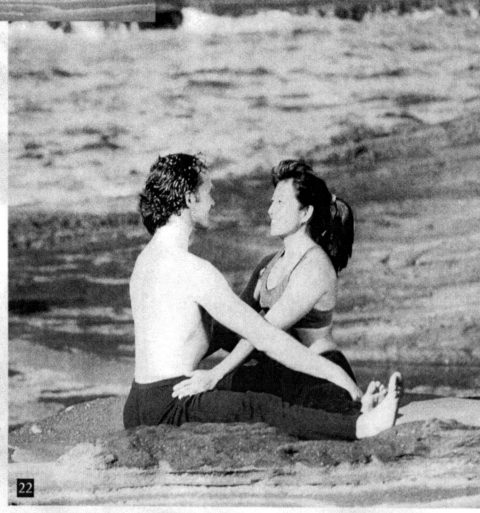
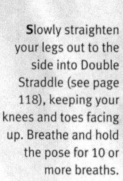

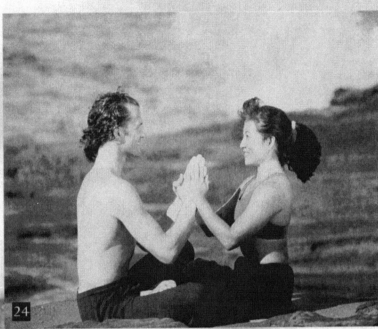

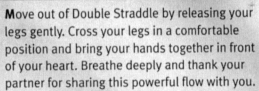

Move out of Double Straddle by releasing your legs gently. Cross your legs in a comfortable position and bring your hands together in front of your heart. Breathe deeply and thank your partner for sharing this powerful flow with you.

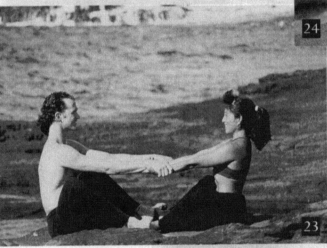

While maintaining hand and foot contact with your partner, bend your knees and scoot toward your partner.

The Relax Flow

The Quick Flow consists of all standing poses, while the Power Flow combines standing and earth poses. In the Relax Flow, all of the poses are practiced on the ground. This is the perfect flow for a quiet evening at home before bed, for a lazy afternoon in the park, or after a long day of work. During this flow, focus on calming your mind and relaxing fully. Let yourself slip into a peaceful space.

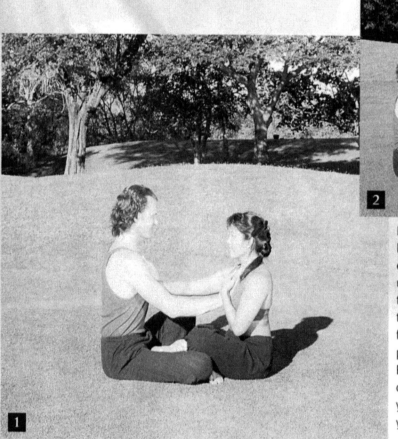

2

Partner One, take Two's hands and begin straightening your legs. Partner Two, unfold your legs and bring the soles of your feet together. One, place your feet on Two's shins and completely straighten your legs. Breathe, relax your shoulders, and lift the crown of your head to the sky. Feel your spine elongate.

1

Begin by sitting cross-legged, facing your partner. Sit close enough to cross your right knee over your partner's left knee and vice versa. Place your right hand over your partner's heart and cover your partner's hand with your left hand. Breathe and connect with your partner. This will set the tone for the rest of the flow.

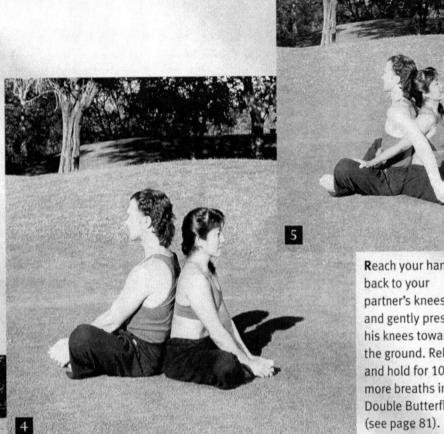

5

4

3

Reach your hands back to your partner's knees and gently press his knees toward the ground. Relax and hold for 10 or more breaths in Double Butterfly (see page 81).

(continued)

Spin gracefully around and sit back to back with your partner. Inhale, lengthen your spine, and bring the soles of your own feet together.

Partner Two, bend forward at your hips into the full Butterfly Forward Bend pose. Partner One, bend forward at your hips and press gently on Two's lower back (see page 80). Hold for 10 or more breaths. Come up slowly and switch positions.

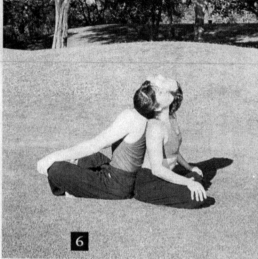

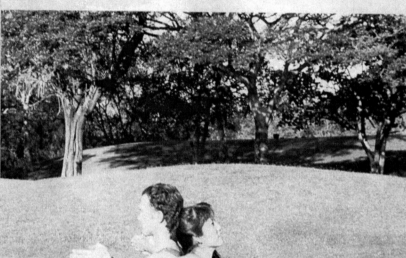

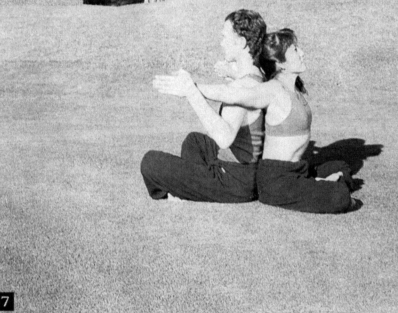

Release your hands and bring your legs into a comfortable cross-legged position. Relax your arms and place them on your own legs. Relax your neck and allow your head to rest on your partner's shoulder. Imagine that you are gazing up at the stars. Hold for about 10 breaths and switch sides.

6

7

Open your arms out to the sides, parallel to the ground. Partner One, reach for Two's hands and gently stretch her arms toward you. Partner Two, breathe and release into the stretch. Explore different angles with your arms to vary the shoulder/chest stretch. Switch roles.

Partner Two, bend forward at
your hips as One brings his knees
together and leans onto your back.

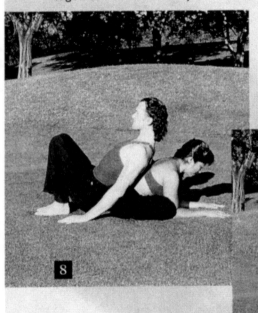

8

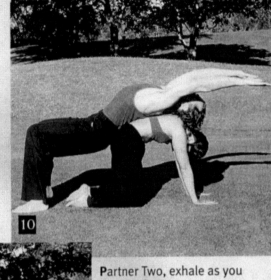

10

Partner Two, exhale as you
press your spine to the sky,
massaging Partner One's spine.
One, bring your arms overhead
to increase your chest and
shoulder stretch.

(continued)

9

Partner Two, push yourself up to your hands and
knees, lifting One onto your back in Massage
Table I (see page 90). One, open your arms out
to the sides, expand your chest, and relax your
entire body.

Partner Two, return to the neutral position, with your back parallel to the ground. Partner One, maintaining back contact, walk your feet around to the side and hang over Two's mid-back for five or more breaths. Return sitting back to back. Switch roles.

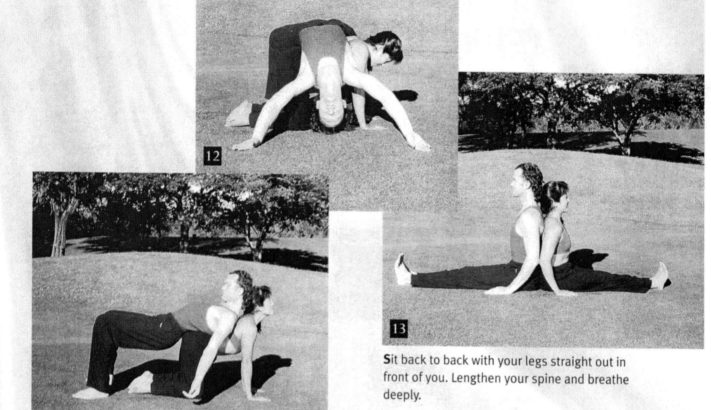

Sit back to back with your legs straight out in front of you. Lengthen your spine and breathe deeply.

Partner Two, inhale as you arch your back, once again massaging One's back. One, relax your arms down to your sides. Alternate in this arching/bowing stretch pattern for four or five rounds.

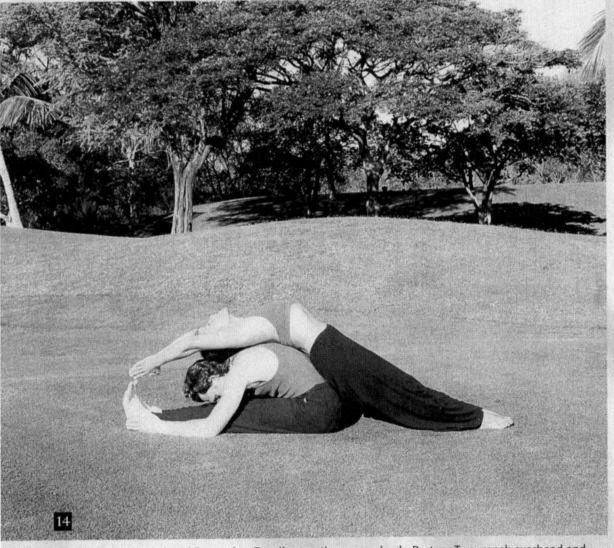

14

Partner One, slowly bend forward as Two lies gently on your back. Partner Two, reach overhead and find One's toes. Help One flex his feet as you arch back into Forward Bend Fish pose (see page 88). Hold for 10 or more breaths. Switch roles.

(continued)

Partner Two, move into the Child pose
(see page 65)and let One lie outstretched
over your back. Relax and hold for 10 or
more breaths. Switch roles.

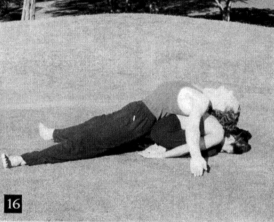

16

Partner One, return to the upright seated position. Partner
Two, squat with your back against Partner One's back.

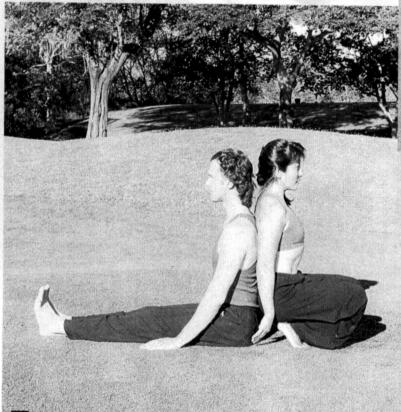

15

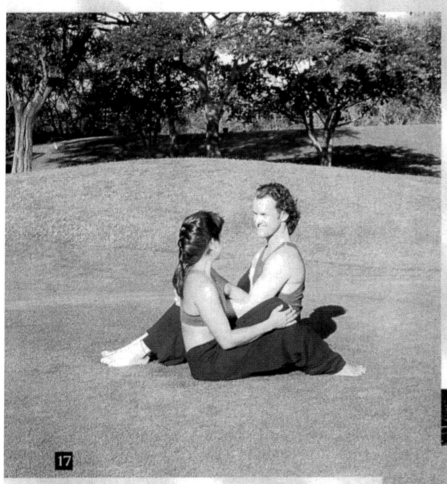

17

Move to the side and back so you are sitting thigh to thigh with your partner. Link inside arms and extend a gesture of appreciation to your partner.

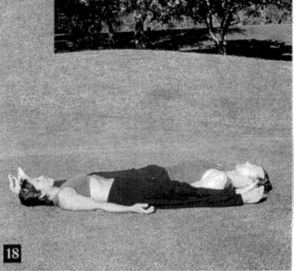

18

Using your partner's arm for support, lower yourself down to Corpse Pose (see page 65), facing opposite directions. Relax for a few minutes before getting up slowly.

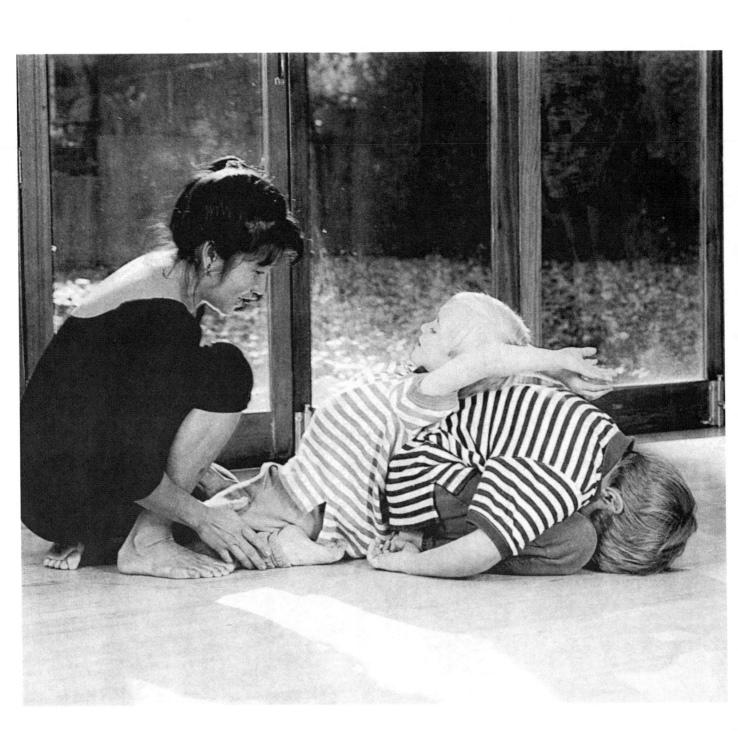

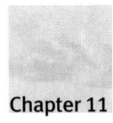

Chapter 11

Making It Personal

"This is your life, and nobody is going to teach you, no book, no guru. You have to learn from yourself, not from books. It is an endless thing, it is a fascinating thing, and when you learn about yourself from yourself, out of that learning wisdom comes."

—J. Krishnamurti, renowned spiritual teacher

Thus far we have presented the basic Partner Yoga philosophy, postures, and flows. These guidelines and suggestions are important tools for learning and growth. They're here to get you started on your journey. Each step of the way we have asked you to look inside yourself and discover what is true for you. By continually paying attention to your unique inner voice, you maximize your benefits and prevent injuries. Staying conscious from moment to moment and knowing how to make the necessary adjustments takes practice. If you notice that you are pushing yourself too hard, do you back off, breathe, and relax? If you are not feeling well or have a specific injury, do you take the extra time to really get in touch with what you need? In this chapter, we present guidelines for working with some of the more common situations that require special attention. Sift through the ideas presented here and see what could be useful specifically for you.

Injuries, Imbalances, or Illnesses

Note: If an injury, imbalance, or illness worsens or persists without improvement, consult an appropriate health professional.

Sciatica and Lower-Back Pain (Lumbago)

Many people complain of dull aches in their lower backs, their buttocks, or the backs of their thighs. The pain worsens with exercise, and sometimes there is periodic sharp pain shooting through the buttocks and down one or both legs. These are common symptoms of sciatica, which comes from stress or pressure somewhere along the sciatic nerve. This nerve starts at the lower back and runs all the way down the back of the leg to the foot. There are myriad causes for sciatica, from tight muscles, chronic spinal misalignment, injury, or a herniated disc to psycho-emotional concerns. Many of the same things that cause sciatica also cause lumbago. In addition, lower-back pain can be caused by weak abdominal muscles or a big belly; foot, ankle, knee, or leg misalignment; neck and shoulder problems; or other causes that are not directly at the site of the pain. We have found yoga to be extremely helpful in preventing or relieving sciatica and lower-back pain. If pain persists, it is always best to consult a professional to address your specific needs.

To stretch out tight muscles after a long run or a session at the gym, postures like **Double Downward Dog** (see page 70) or **Downward Dog Back Bend** (see page 72) are great. The Downward Dog posture stretches out the hips and legs. In addition, **Double Triangle** (see page 106) or **Double Revolved Triangle** (see page 108) work on stretching the hip in rotation, which people with sciatica and lumbago often need. Seated forward bends (see pages 79, 80, and 88) stretch the buttocks and lower back, with the focus on lengthening the spine. **Rising Cobra** (see page 114) and **Child Camel** (see page 126) can tonify the entire spine and correct misalignments.

For more advanced yogis, hold **The Backpack** variation (see page 103) for a few minutes, or practice any of the lifts that allow your back to hang or stretch in a bow position. These are excellent ways to allow the back to find its natural alignment. If you have an acute strain, the smartest thing to do is, of course, *rest*. Once again, go slowly and listen carefully to your body. Always breathe deeply and relax into postures without tension or strain.

Neck and Shoulder Pain

As with lower-back pain and sciatica, neck and shoulder pain can be caused by many different things. Treatment depends on whether your pain is acute or chronic. If the pain is acute—from an injury or acute misalignment of some sort—usually the best thing to do is rest and practice deep breathing exercises. Resting postures such as **Child Pose** or **Corpse Pose** (see page 65) are helpful.

Lori: *Eight years ago, I had a serious injury to my neck. While crossing the street, I was hit by a car and broke my neck in nine places. There were multiple fractures in three vertebrae and bone fragments impinging nerves in the nerve canals. Neurosurgeons suggested neck surgery, yet my intuitive voice said otherwise. With rest, a soft neck brace, deep breathing exercises, visualization, gentle yoga stretches, and some good naturopathic and chiropractic help, the repeat CT scan showed all the fractures had healed within 6 months, and the bone fragments had migrated back into alignment.*

Chronic neck and shoulder problems are usually due to postural strain or repetitive work conditions such as computer or telephone jobs—or perhaps the "responsibilities of life" weighing too heavily on your shoulders. **Downward Dog** poses (see pages 70 and 72) held for a few minutes relieve stiffness in the shoulders and open up the upper back. **The M Bend** (see page 139) provides a good stretch for tight shoulders. If you need something more gentle, the arm stretch in the **Relax Flow** (see page 186) can be a gentler way to increase shoulder range of motion. One of the best postures for relieving neck and shoulder pain is **Hanging Forward Bend** (see page 152). Hanging in this position for 5 to 10 minutes, with your partner helping you relax your shoulders, can make you feel like you are floating on cloud nine.

For advanced yogis, **Lifted Bow** (see page 156) and **Lifted Camel** (see page 160) really open the upper back, shoulders, and neck. Hold postures for a few extra minutes (as long as you aren't creating more strain) to allow your muscles to relax and release long-stored tension. Once again, if pain persists, consult a professional.

Headaches

Headaches are becoming as pervasive as the common cold. Headaches come from muscular tightness, mental pressure, vascular irregularities, food allergies, toxins, and a wide array of other things.

Note: Seek professional help immediately if headaches are recurrent in children or the elderly, if they occur suddenly and severely without prior history, or if they are associated with high fever, convulsions, head trauma, loss of consciousness, or localized pain in the ear, eye, or elsewhere.

The following yoga postures are helpful for headaches that are related to stress, muscle tension, or poor circulation. **Partner Shoulderstand** (see page

124) regulates the supply of blood to the head by its firm chin lock. If the pose is held for 5 to 10 minutes, the nerves are soothed and even chronic headaches disappear. This pose also stimulates your thyroid and parathyroid glands, located in your neck, regulating metabolism and calming your entire body. If Partner Shoulderstand is too difficult, **Partner Plow** (see page 123) has similar effects. Hold this posture for 3 to 5 minutes to achieve the best results.

Believe it or not, standing on your head can also help to relieve many headaches. The headstand is known as the father of all postures, and it brings healthy, pure blood and fresh oxygen to the brain cells. Refer to the work-up photos for **Double Scorpion** (see page 144) for help in getting up into a headstand. Practice a modified version of **Yin Yang Handstand** (see page 142). Instead of a handstand, get up into a headstand and have your partner support you in the same way as for Yin Yang Handstand. If standing on your head seems just a little too energetic, simple postures like **The Table** (see page 68), **Hanging Forward Bend** (see page 152), or resting postures with deep breathing (see pages 64 and 65) often calm the mind enough to relieve headaches.

Allergies and Sinus Problems

We have probably all had a runny nose sometime in our lives. Increasing mucus is just the body's way of getting rid of wastes or toxins. Sometimes, though, our bodies can start reacting to everything from dust, mold, and pollens to foods, smells, and toxins in the air. When this happens, it's helpful to strengthen the immune system and minimize mucus-producing foods. Breathing techniques (see chapter 4) and specific nostril breathing (see books on Pranayama in the bibliography on page 232) keep the nasal passages clear.

Try postures that open the chest, expand the lungs, and tonify the entire respiratory system, such as **Child Camel** (see page 126) and **Heart Opener** (see page 128). Although they may initially accelerate the mucus flow, inversions increase circulation to the head and nasal passages, bringing fresh blood to the irritated mucous membranes. If postures are held for at least a few minutes, sinuses start to clear. If your head is too congested, you might need to wait until some of the congestion decreases to practice inversions.

Specific postures such as **Partner Shoulderstand** (see page 124) are excellent for sinus problems or allergies. Both positions in this partner posture are beneficial, since sometimes we simply need to sit and align in order for our breathing passages to open up. **Double Seated Forward Bend** (see page 79) and standing forward bends such as in **The Backpack** (see page 102) are also helpful.

Fatigue

Many people come to our yoga classes to generate more energy. They come stressed and tired and leave feeling lifted and energetic. A Partner Yoga session can be like a good overall tonic.

If you are tired, it can be helpful to identify the source of your fatigue. You might ask yourself, "Am I working too hard? How's my stress level? Is my thyroid gland working okay? Am I sleeping well? How's my circulation? Am I getting enough exercise, fun, and nourishment in my life? Could I have a chronic virus?" By identifying the source of your fatigue, you will be able to choose Partner Yoga postures that address your specific needs. Consulting a health professional for a specific plan is also a good idea.

Inversions like **Partner Plow** and **Partner Shoulderstand** (see pages 123 and 124) relieve fatigue by stimulating the thyroid and parathyroid glands and tonifying the endocrine and nervous systems. Downward dog postures (see pages 70 and 72) bring healthy blood to the brain without straining the heart. Standing forward bends, as in **The Backpack** (see page 102) or **The Table** (see page 68), calm the mind if they're held for more than a couple of minutes. Often, fatigue comes from the mind as well as the body. The **Massage Table** postures (see pages 90 and 92) and resting postures (see pages 64 and 65) are also specifically designed to relieve both mental and physical fatigue.

Yoga for Women
During a Woman's Cycle: Menstruation

Since a woman's body changes during menstruation, it is a perfect opportunity to tune in a little more carefully. Some women feel like taking a break from Partner Yoga during this time and spending more time alone. Others find that yoga can enhance bloodflow and body cleansing. The most important thing is to be sensitive to your changing needs.

It is best to avoid abdominal lifts or abdominal strengthening exercises like leg lifts or situps. Inversions are not suggested. During menstruation, nature wants the energy to go down and out, and inversion postures draw the energy up.

Double Downward Dog (see page 70), **The Pump** (see page 74), and **Standing Straddle** (see page 76) are fine with minimal holding. Extreme back bending can actually stop menstrual flow because of the intense pressure on the vertebrae near the pelvic girdle. On the other hand, moderate back bending opens the abdominal and pelvic areas and relieves menstrual discomfort.

Forward bending postures like **Double Seated Forward Bend** (see page 79) or **Butterfly Forward Bend** (see page 80) massage the pelvic organs. Both positions in **Forward Bend Fish** (see page 88) are excellent for menstruation. If you need a support when bending forward, relax your belly into a soft pillow. Performing the **Rising Cobra** (see page 114) with a pillow under your belly also gives you a good pelvic and abdominal massage.

Pregnancy

Pregnancy is an amazing adventure and a time of great change. Your body, mind, emotions, and spirit are engaged in the process of creating a new life. Partner Yoga is perfect for this time of shifting focus. Partner Yoga cultivates a strong and supportive environment in which to raise a child. In the photo below, the couple is practicing **Double Straddle** (see page 118), which opens the heart along with the hips.

In the early stages of pregnancy, you can do almost any of the postures as long

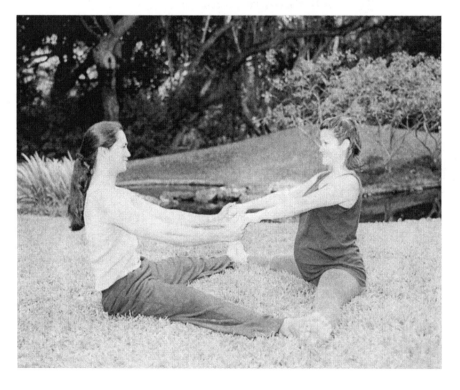

as you don't strain and don't hold postures for long. Lift postures and spinal twists are best avoided throughout pregnancy. Naturally, be extremely careful with any posture that puts pressure on the pelvic area or abdomen. During the first 12 weeks of pregnancy, nourishment, rest, deep breathing, a few gentle stretches, and playfulness is what we most recommend. Once you are in your second trimester, you can add more postures to your Partner Yoga routine. Still, you don't ever want to jerk or strain when going in or out of postures.

To increase spinal flexibility and make more room for your baby, practice the **Massage Table I and II** (see pages 90 and 92) and a modified version of **The Fountain** without a deep back bend (see page 98). These postures are gentle, yet they really get the spine moving. **The Porthole** (see page 110) stretches your back, hips, and legs. For increasing hip flexibility, **Double Butterfly** (see page 81) and squatting are excellent. In the photo to the right, two pregnant moms play with a new posture we call **Double Squat**. It opens the hips and legs while working on balance and mutual support.

Other balance postures such as **Double Tree** (see page 133) and **Standing Star** (see page 134) also benefit pregnancy by im-

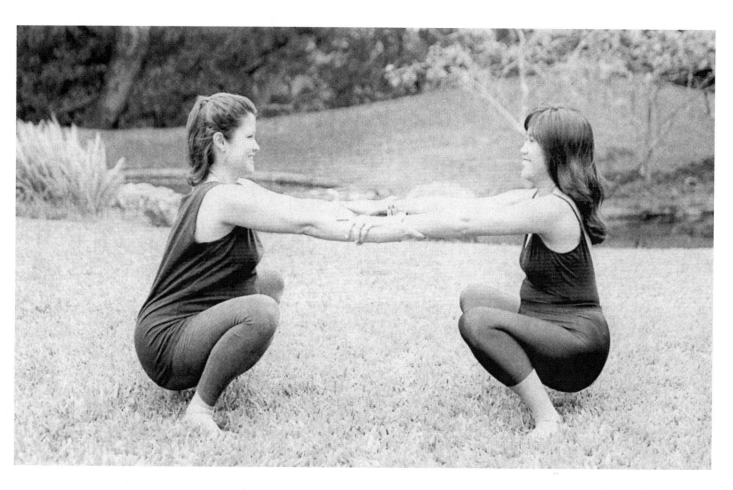

proving circulation and steadying the mind. The calming influence of balance poses will be helpful throughout pregnancy and during labor. Whichever postures you choose to do, though, remember that pregnancy is first and foremost a time for rest and nourishment.

Parents and Kids

Kids grow up so fast. One day, they're playing on their swings, and the next time you turn around, they're roaring off in some fancy car. Spending quality time with them when they're young is essential. All along, we have emphasized how Partner Yoga enriches relationships. A parent-child relationship is no exception. Share the principles of Partner Yoga with your kids. Make games out of postures, like getting them to act out the characteristics of the animal that a posture represents. They can bark like a dog in **Downward Dog** poses (see page 70) or hiss like a cobra in **Rising Cobra** (see page 114) or **Lifted Cobra** (see page 148). Let your own inner child come out and play. Modify poses depending on what you think your child would enjoy. In the photo below, Mom is adding movement to the **Lifted Back Bend** pose (see page 154), swinging her daughter gently back and forth and adding to her fun.

Poses that involve climbing or lifting are fun for adventurous children. **Double Downward Dog** (see page 70), **The Backpack** (see page 102), **Two Scoops** (see page 122), **Lifted Cobra** (see page 148), or any of the lifts (see chapter 9) are fun to play with. If your child is not quite as daring, start simply with a modified **Rising Cobra** (see page 114) or **Double Straddle** (see page 118). Most kids love **Hanging Forward Bend** (see page 152) so much that they'll ask for it again and again.

Kid Stuff

Starting yoga at a young age gives children a strong foundation for the rest of their lives. Yoga reinforces their natural flexibility and sense of balance and cultivates their ability to focus. Practicing Partner Yoga exposes children to the principles of mutual support, sharing, and effective communication. They experience the benefits of working with, rather than fighting against, another person. Most kids are naturally adventurous and want to have fun. They are also naturally touch-oriented, and Partner Yoga is an excellent way to extend their comfort with physical contact as they grow up. If you simply let them play, kids get into all kinds of partner postures on their own. It is inspiring to watch their

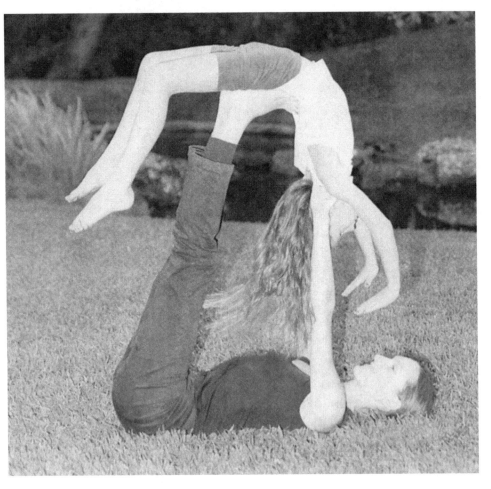

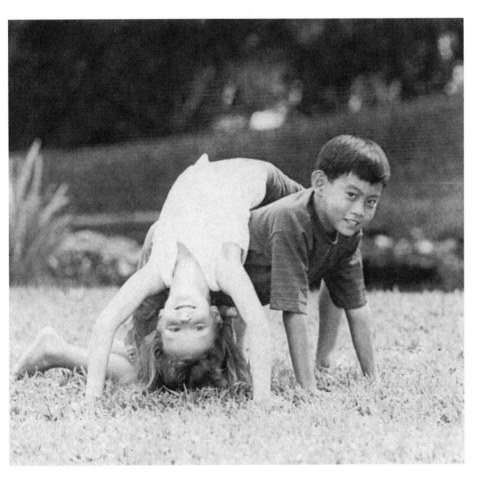

keep their attention. In our photo shoot, the two kids in the photo to the left, who hadn't met before, had lots of fun and became friends after just a couple of poses.

Looking Forward

Ultimately, everything requires special consideration. Your internal and external environment is changing all the time. By now, you probably understand why we con-

creativity flow, uninhibited by the restraints of adult society.

Playful postures that kids love to practice are **Double Chair** (see page 69), **Double Downward Dog** (see page 70), **Forward Bend Fish** (see page 88), **Massage Table I and II** (see pages 90 and 92), **Double Boat** (see page 116), **Two Scoops** (see page 122), and **Double Tree** (see page 133). Since children often have short attention spans, these poses are easily made into fun games to

tinually say to "go inside yourself and see what is true for you." After all, you do know yourself best, and you are your own best teacher. We can only help to guide you back to yourself. It is best to ask yourself first and then get support as needed. As you tap into that infinite source of wisdom deep inside of you, your truth becomes clearer and your life unfolds with greater ease. Fasten your seatbelts—the journey has just begun.

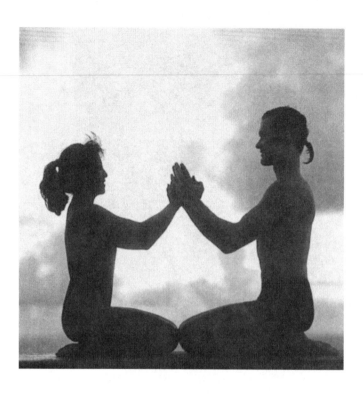

PART THREE

EXPANDING BEYOND

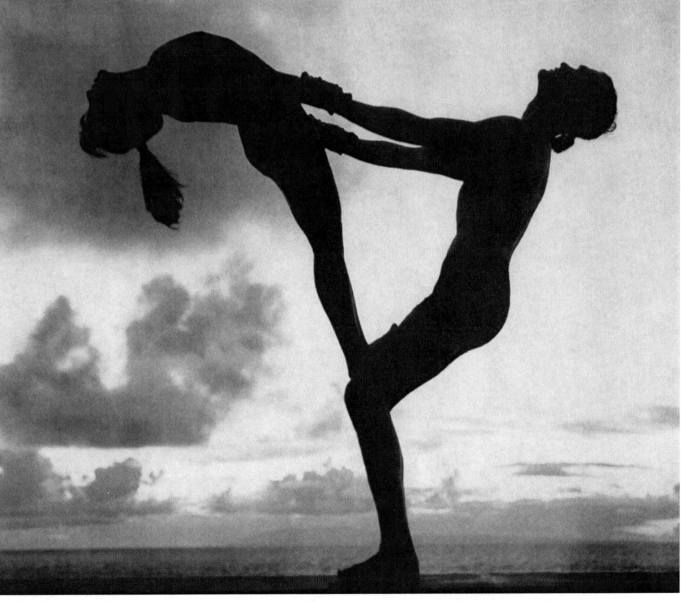

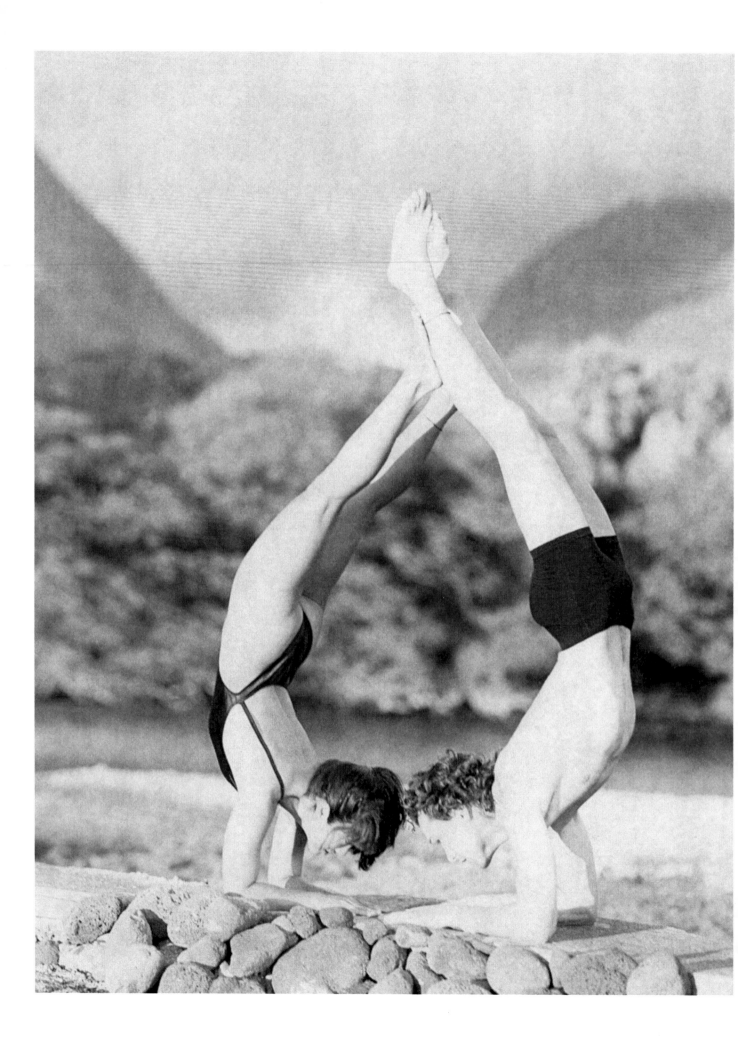

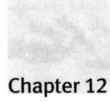

Chapter 12

Mindful Courage

"Courage is a clean, simple virtue. It is powered by love. It declares to the world, 'I love this person or thing or idea so much that I will risk for it.'"

—Edward J. Lavin, S.J., author of *Life Meditations*

Courage. When you read that word, what comes to mind? Many people associate courage with the heroic feats of soldiers, firefighters, mountain climbers, or other brave souls who risk their health or even their lives. Indeed, it takes great courage to confront the fear of death, enter a burning building, or ascend an icy peak, and those who do certainly stand among us as heroes. The deeds of many of our heroes, however, are not so visible: the mother who nurtures a child, the man who tells the truth, the person who learns to forgive, the child who tries something new. Courage is expressed in many ways. This chapter is about exploring the subtle inner nature of what it means to be courageous.

Let's cut right to the core. If we are going to talk about courage, we have to take a look at its closest cousins, fear and pain. Courage usually takes form in the face of fear, and fear takes form in the face of pain. For humans, pain is a basic experience. It begins at birth and continues, to some degree or another, intermittently throughout our lives. We are continually learning about pain. Pain manifests in many ways, and each person experiences pain in a different way. Some people live with physical pain from injuries, chronic tension, or on-going discomfort from a condition such as arthritis. Others experience pain on a mental-emotional level, living with sadness, loneliness, resentment, or jealousy.

Fear exists because pain is real. Essentially, fear is a sensation that we experience when we are confronted with the possibility of feeling pain. Since each of us experiences pain differently, we are all afraid of different things and react in different ways. For example, consider the following two scenarios.

A firefighter arrives at the location of a burning home. Flames have engulfed the house, and the roof is beginning to cave in. There is a good chance that someone is stuck in one of the back rooms. The firefighter feels a surge of fear as she is uncertain of how much time she has until the whole house collapses, and the possibility of being burned or crushed is horrifying.

A new sales associate is traveling with his boss to an annual conference to assist in the presentation of their company's new line of products. During the flight, his boss becomes very ill, and upon landing, he has to be hospitalized. The conference begins in 2 hours, and it looks as if the new associate is going to have to take his boss's place in representing the company. Upon realizing this, the associate is overtaken by fear. He has never led a presentation of this

magnitude, and the thought of speaking by himself in front of hundreds of industry leaders causes him to feel nauseated and dizzy. His greatest fear is appearing unprepared or inept in the eyes of his peers.

In each of these scenarios, the characters are confronted with feeling pain. Although the nature of the pain is entirely different, the threat of pain produces the same response in both: fear. At this point, each has numerous options. If the firefighter acts consciously, there is a better chance that she will be able to safely rescue the trapped person. Similarly, if the associate meets his fear head on, he can convert this fear into an energy that can be used in his presentation.

This brings us back to the notion of courage. In both of these scenarios, the best possible outcome occurs when fear is met with awareness. The ability to stay totally present in that moment of fear is what we call mindful courage.

The Now: Our Final Frontier

As you delve deeper into the practice of Partner Yoga, you will inevitably cross the path of fear and pain. Admittedly, your experience in Partner Yoga probably will not be as intense as that of the imaginary characters mentioned above. However, the opportunity to practice mindful courage is present. In many

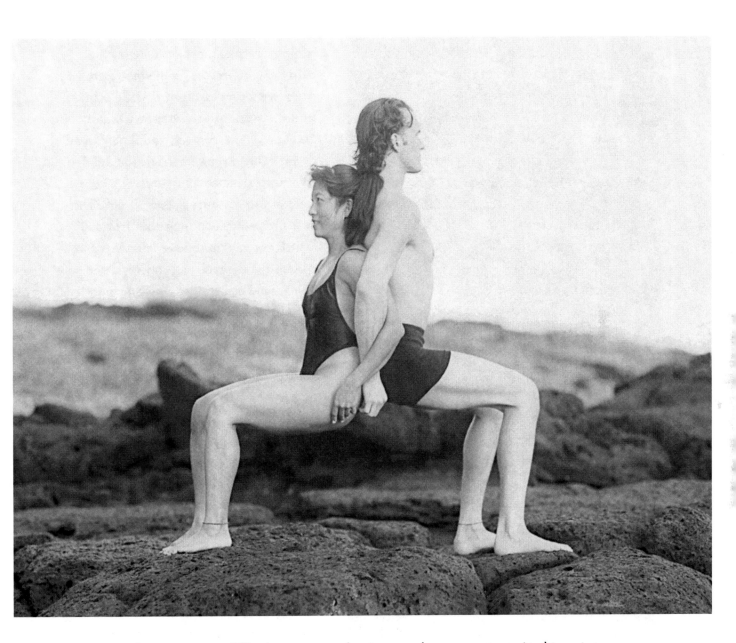

ways, it may be even more difficult to practice mindful courage in a situation where the fear is less intense. For example, imagine that you and a new partner are taking a moment to tune in before warming up (see page 46). Your hands are in partner namaste and you

begin to make eye contact. At this point, you feel a little vulnerable, and after a couple of seconds, you shift your eyes and sort of "check out"—the interaction is just too intimate.

This scenario is actually very common in Partner Yoga. Let's break it down. Say

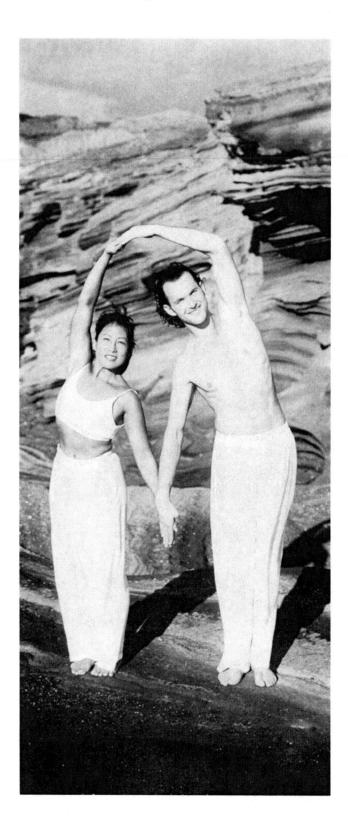

that your intention was to connect with your partner to practice some partner poses and experience something new. You knew the poses involved physical contact, and you were okay with that. Up until the moment of eye contact, you thought you were feeling pretty open and uninhibited. When you caught your partner's eye, a part of you instantly slammed shut. The fear of possibly exposing your true self was a little too much. If this person caught a glimpse of the real you, she might see your foibles and insecurities. And the emotional pain of rejection was something you would rather avoid altogether. The possibility of experiencing this pain produced the feeling of fear. In turn, the conditioned reaction was to run the other way.

Practicing mindful courage in a situation like this can be quite challenging. First, you must observe the subtle undulations of your thoughts and feelings. Second, you have to stay so keenly aware of the moment that you avoid the rut of conditioned reaction; this requires you to bring consciousness to each of your actions. And finally, you must find the strength to stand up to your fears. The strength required to confront this kind of fear comes from accepting your true self, and the fuel for that acceptance is Love.

Traversing Boundaries

In our experience with Partner Yoga, we have found that many of our limitations are self-imposed. Oftentimes, these limitations are a result of how we deal with fear. Sometimes we notice feelings of fear during intense hamstring stretches (such as Forward Bend Fish), and other times they surface while practicing lift poses (like Lifted Lotus). There is nothing wrong with this fear. Feeling fear is completely natural. What we have learned is that if we run from our fear or allow fear to control us, we have limited our experience. If we simply meet fear in the moment, it has no hold on us.

Our most memorable experiences in Partner Yoga are those when we found the strength to traverse the boundaries of our fears. It did not happen by brute force or by convincing ourselves that we were not afraid. It happened when, in the yoga of the moment, we were truly practicing mindful courage. As you take your own practice further, we challenge you to continually confront your fears, to be honest with yourself and your partner, and to trust that with mindful courage each moment will unfold perfectly.

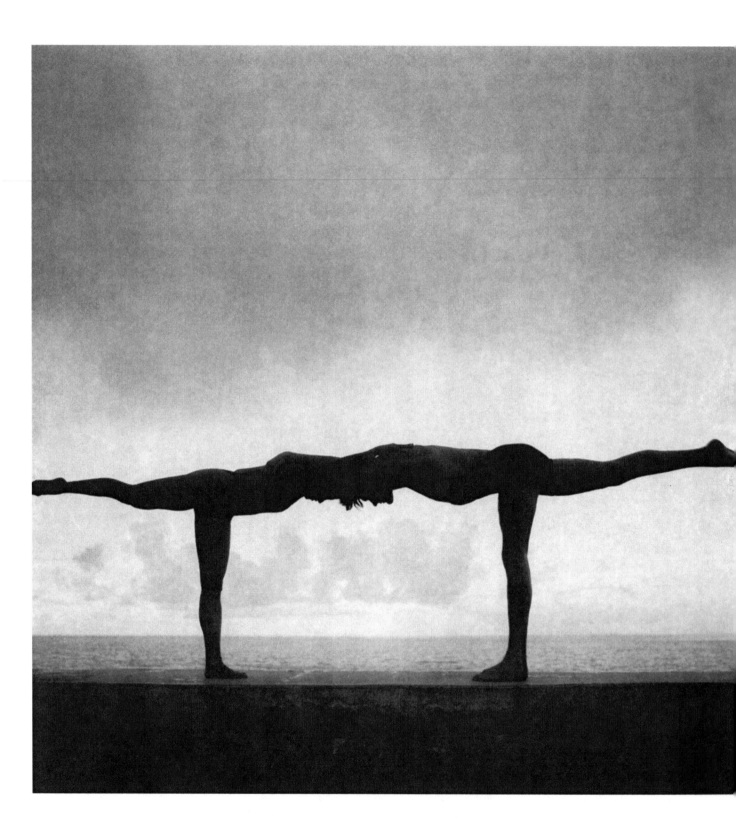

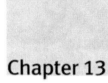

Chapter 13

Create Your Own Dance

"The creative is the place where no one else has ever been. You have to leave the city of your comfort and go into the wilderness of your intuition. You can't get there by bus, only by hard work, risk, and not quite knowing what you're doing. What you discover will be quite wonderful. What you'll discover will be yourself."

—Alan Alda

The real beauty of Partner Yoga is making it your own unique practice. You now have the basic tools. You know the importance of breath, alignment, and warming up. You have a repertoire of basic postures and variations, and you understand the implications behind them. Now it's time to put it all together, to venture out into new territory, to go somewhere that you have never been.

We are all creative beings. You don't have to be a clever artist or have years of experience, you just need to show up! You are creative just by being you. You are an absolute original, and whatever you do that comes from your true self is absolutely unique. As contemporary philosopher Frank Gonzales simply put it, "Sure, the wheel has been created before, but it has never been created by me."

We are here to live and express fully all the unique wonders that lie within us.

Creativity has no limits. It begins with realizing that you are freer than you think. Richard Bach puts it well in his bestseller *Jonathan Livingston Seagull*, where he tells the story of a gull named Jonathan who learns what unlimited freedom really means. Jonathan tells the other gulls, "You have the freedom to be yourself, your true self, here and now, and nothing can stand in your way—freedom is the very nature of your being." For seagulls and humans alike, Jonathan's statement is altogether true. If you want to soar, you have to start by spreading your wings.

A Creative Exercise: The Dancer and the Universe

Let's dive headfirst into an exercise that will expand your creative mind/body. This exercise is based on a training technique used by Butoh dancers. Butoh is a dance form that combines meditation, improvisation, and the use of a technique called following. The purpose of this exercise is to practice letting go of the rational mind, while learning to follow the subtle signals of your intuition, your environment, and your partner. As your awareness grows, you will be able to access your reservoir of creativity with less effort. This exploration takes about 10 minutes, and it's best done in an open space where you can move

about freely without the fear of running into things.

The Beginning

Begin by designating one partner to be the Dancer and the other the Universe. Stand facing your partner about a foot apart. Bring your palms together at your heart and acknowledge your partner with a smile. Release your hands to your sides and relax your shoulders. Close your eyes, quiet your mind, and still your body. Tune in to your breathing and feel how your body expands and contracts with each breath. Begin to take note of how the weight of your body balances over your feet. Notice how although your body feels still, your balance is not static. Instead, your balance is the result of a dynamic process involving a continuous series of slight adjustments. Focus even deeper, and feel how your body sways from side to side and how your weight shifts over your feet. Now let go of the idea of actively holding your body still, and simply allow yourself to experience the dynamics of balance as if you were watching yourself from above. Take about 3 minutes to complete this exercise.

The Exploration

Dancer, throughout all of this exploration, your eyes will remain closed; this is integral to the exploration (if you think you might cheat, use a blindfold). Universe, slowly open your eyes and walk to the

Dancer's left side. With your right hand, reach to the little finger on her left hand, lightly holding only the tip between your thumb and forefinger. Breathe.

Dancer, bring all of your awareness to the tip of your left little finger. Imagine that your rational mind is shutting off and that your little finger has taken its place in perceiving reality. Feel as though your little finger is responsible for guiding your every move. Surrender your entire being to your little finger, and follow its guidance without question (here is where the fun begins).

Universe, slowly begin to lead the Dancer by her little finger in any direction you feel. Allow yourself to move freely without thinking. Take the dancer up to the sky and down to the floor, and around and about with no rhyme or reason, varying the pace of your movement. Dancer, your only job is to follow the Universe without hesitation or judgment.

Take about 7 minutes to complete the exploration. Then switch roles and repeat from the beginning.

The Birth of a New Partner Pose

There was a gentle breeze blowing on the south shore of

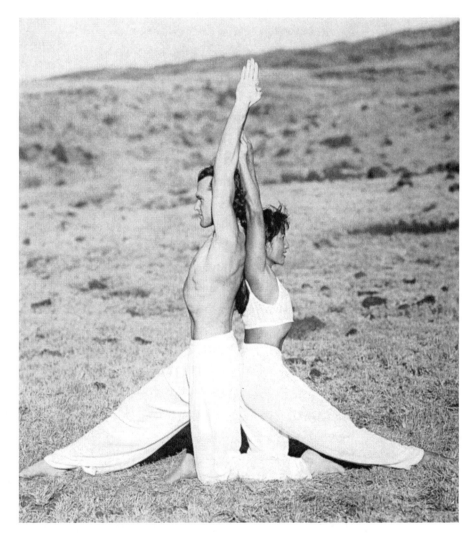

Maui as we piled out of our traveling studio to catch the first rays of sun. We were at the beginning of another exciting day of photo shooting. We took a few moments to connect and honor each other, our group, and the beautiful emerging day. We knelt in the grass and let ourselves play, much like we had the first time we made contact years ago in Phoenix. We had driven quite a while to get to our sunrise destination, and we needed something to open up our chests and backs, stretch our arms and shoulders, massage our buttocks, and give our legs a gentle wake-up call. We cleared our minds, connected our hearts, made physical contact, and started spontaneously stretching. The environment and mood were just perfect for creativity. Within a few minutes, we found ourselves in a totally new posture together—something neither of us had ever seen or done before. We call this new posture The Steeple (see page 146).

To get your creative juices flowing, do at least one new thing every day for 3 weeks as an experiment. It doesn't matter what you do; anything will work. Here are some examples we've done in the past: Take a different route to work; wear a color you normally don't wear; open doors with your nondominant hand; enter an elevator and stand with your back to the door, observing and smiling at your fellow passengers. The point is to create a shift in perspective and allow yourself to stretch beyond your usual paradigm. Start simple and expand from there. Creativity begets creativity.

Get Lost

We continue to surprise each other—and ourselves—in our partner practice. After moving spontaneously, we'll find ourselves in a new posture and wonder how we got there. There are other times that we struggle, coming up with only strange contortions of no real benefit. We have accepted that in exploring new territory, we can easily get lost along the way.

We remember the first time we practiced a lift posture. Our initial fear gave way to an exhilarating feeling of accomplishment as we secured the new posture. The keys to executing a beautiful lift are patience, mindful trial and error, and a light sense of humor. Success comes with patience and the willingness to go places we haven't gone before.

Lori: *As a kid, I was really good at copying. I would watch other people's behavior to discover which actions were rewarded and which were frowned upon. Anxious for approval, I knew just what dance to do to please everyone. It wasn't "my" dance; it was the dance that worked. It seemed to get me what I thought I wanted at the time. One day many years later, I caught myself doing that same dance I used as a kid to please my parents. I took a deep breath to get some perspective. I had been dancing other people's dances for so long, I had forgotten that they weren't my own. As Ralph Waldo Emerson reminds me, "Insist on yourself; never imitate. Your own gift you can present every moment with the cumulative force of a whole life's cultivation."*

Enhancing Creativity

If you have practiced yoga before, experiment with traditional posture combinations that are mutually supportive. If you aren't familiar with traditional yoga postures, let your body, mind, emotions, and spirit guide you. Maybe today you feel the need to address fear and want to play with back bending. Maybe your calves are tight and you can create a partner posture that will help to loosen them. You don't have to produce some fabulous new posture, just a simple variation will do. If you are practicing one of the flows, how about adding one or two partner postures in between, at the beginning, or at the end?

Experiment with practicing Partner Yoga in different environments. If you are used to practicing indoors, find a space outdoors to practice. The change of environment might stir your creativity. On one of those 110°F days in Phoenix, we jumped into a pool and started playing with Partner Yoga. Within a few hours, we had almost enough new postures for another book on "Pool Partner Yoga"! To give our feet a break from the rocks during our

photo shoot, we suddenly jumped into a sandy tide pool and created a new experience with one of our familiar postures.

Practicing Partner Yoga with a couple of friends or even a group of friends adds another creative dimension. Sometimes there are three of you who want to practice together, and finding postures that you can all do together is challenging and fun. We stumbled into the new group posture below during our photo shoot. Half the fun is not having any idea of what is going to happen and

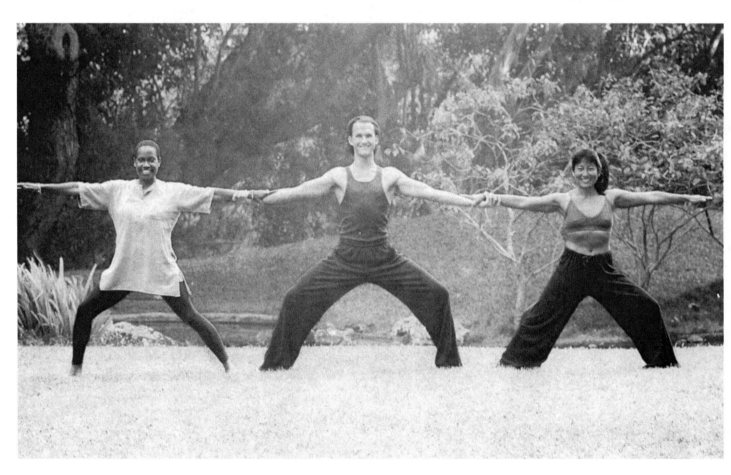

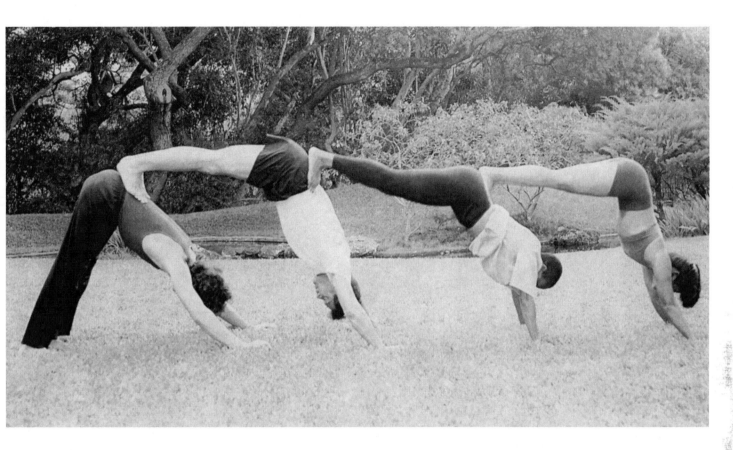

letting it all unfold. In this spontaneous group posture, we're all getting a leg workout, a great arm stretch, and a grin from ear to ear, especially the guy in the middle.

Then another of our friends came along and we found a way to integrate him into our fun as well. Adding two more people into the original Double Downward Dog creates a fun new dynamic. You will be amazed at what you can conjure up with combined creativity and effective group communication.

Create your own Partner Yoga postures and flows and share them with others. The Partner Yoga playground is a wide open space.

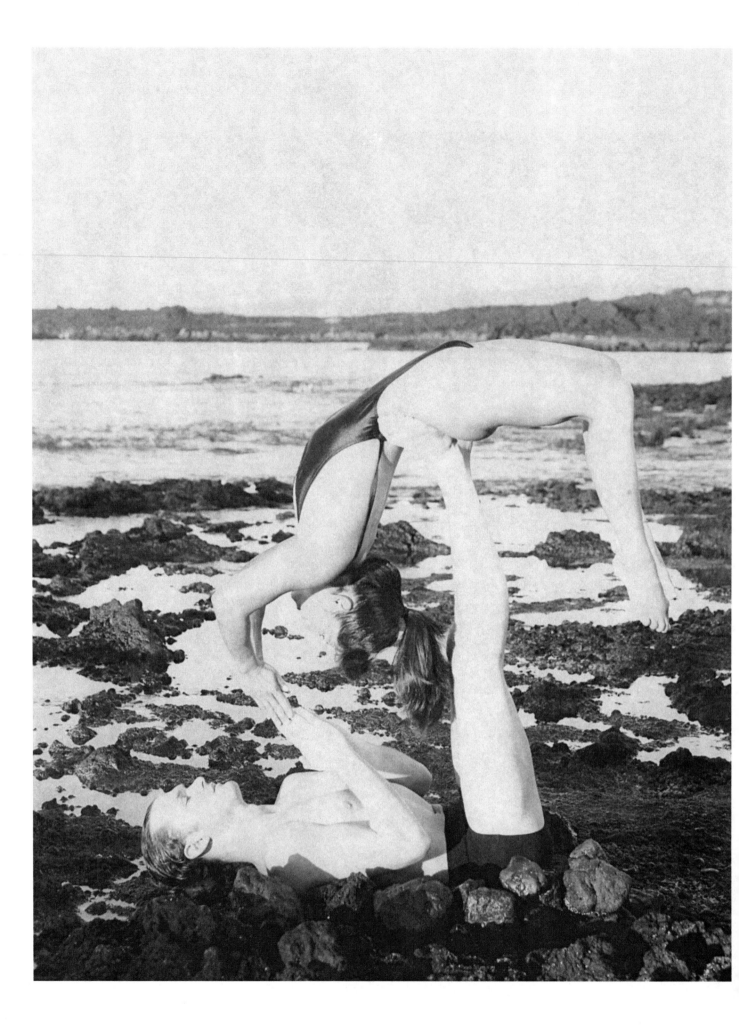

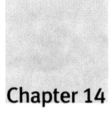

Chapter 14

Intimacy

"Pare down to the essence, but don't remove the poetry."

—Leonard Koren, author of *Wabi-Sabi for Artists, Designers, Poets, and Philosophers*

We come into the world naked and vulnerable. Over time, most of us get the message that the world is a scary place and protection is necessary. We build a wide array of defenses, and before long, the naked, vulnerable child is well-hidden. Intimacy is about peeling away those defensive layers and getting in touch with our true selves. Imagine peeling the layers of an onion. You peel away the tougher outer layers to get to the softer, more tender layers, and sometimes you shed a few tears. So it is with intimacy. With the release of each layer, a more tender part of yourself is exposed. This process is not always easy, but it's what Partner Yoga is all about. Embracing intimacy involves awareness of breath, alignment, strength, stamina, flexibility, trust, surrender, balance, grace, and mindful courage. In short, everything we've presented in this book was created with the intention of embracing intimacy.

Getting Rid of Your Intimacy Armor

In the charming book *The Knight in Rusty Armor*, Robert Fisher tells the story of an archetypal knight who gets stuck in his armor. No one can touch him, nor can he touch anyone. He can't even feel his own skin. His armor keeps him from feeling much of anything. He almost forgets how it feels to be

221

free. The process of getting rid of his armor is long and challenging. The knight learns that he had put on his armor to shut out the world because he was afraid and he thought the armor would keep him protected. He discovers that the armor kept him from himself as well. In the end,

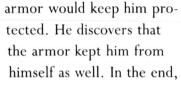

his heart opens, his burden is released, and he goes inward on his path of truth.

Like the knight in the story, many of us have developed mechanisms to protect ourselves and separate us from the world. Some of these mechanisms, like the knight's armor, are easy to see. Others are so well-concealed that we hardly even know they're there. Practicing Partner Yoga gives you the opportunity to look at your armor. Are you comfortable peeling off a few protective layers? After all, Partner Yoga does involve physical contact. Are you able and willing to express your feelings and your needs? What kind of intimacy armor do you have that keeps you from being more intimate with yourself or other people?

A Panoramic View of Intimacy

The word "intimacy" comes from the root word "intima," which means the innermost structure of something. In our culture, intimacy is often associated with sexual intimacy. Although this is one important aspect of intimacy, there are other aspects as well. Intimacy can be experienced on many levels— emotional, mental, physical, and spiritual. Take pen pals or cyber-friends, for example, who share the personal details of life with each other. On a mental/emotional level, they can feel like they know each other very well, although they have never met face-to-face. They have not experienced any form of physical intimacy, yet they feel intimately connected. You might share a deep spiritual connection with someone without sharing your personal life and without any form of physical contact, yet you are experiencing intimacy. Or maybe you have a buddy with whom you cuddle and exchange bodywork, yet you don't have a sexual relationship with that person. And perhaps, in a sexual partnership, you experience the wonder of physical intimacy as it blends with all the other aspects of intimacy.

Feelings of intimacy often get interpreted as feelings of sexual intimacy. Our culture feeds this confusion by promoting sexual intimacy almost exclusively. Therefore, when we want to express intimacy, we often turn to sex. By limiting ourselves to sexual intimacy, however, we are missing out on a whole spectrum of human experience.

If we want to fully embrace life, it is time we widen our view of what it means to be intimate. Partner Yoga provides an opportunity to explore all channels of intimate expression. When you are practicing postures together and feelings of intimacy surface, take a moment to really explore these feelings. Making a deeper, more intimate connection with someone is the intent of Partner Yoga. The most important thing is to become more conscious of how you relate to feelings of intimacy.

When you start a Partner Yoga session, bring awareness to your breath first, and check in with your mind, your heart, and your spirit. Then contact your partner. Feel his breath, feel the touch of his hand on your heart, and gaze gently into his eyes. Looking into someone's eyes immediately gives you the opportunity to feel how comfortable you are with intimacy.

Certain postures can bring up feelings of vulnerability more than others. **Double Straddle**, for example (see page 118), brings you into a close face-to-face posture with your partner. Physical closeness tends to make us feel more intimate. You and your partner can design your Partner Yoga practice to best fit both of your needs.

If you are practicing Partner Yoga with your child, take advantage of this wonderful opportunity to practice intimacy. Honestly sharing who you are with your children is not always easy. Many parents have high standards of how they need to be in front of their kids. Being willing to open your heart, honestly share, and really listen creates intimacy. Remember that true intimacy involves surrendering on its deepest level.

Practicing Partner Yoga is the journey of trekking deeper into the territories of your body, mind, heart, and soul. Setting your own pace makes the adventure much more enjoyable. As you explore feelings of trust, surrender, fear, and intimacy, stay conscious and act truthfully. Most important, have fun, laugh as much as possible, and practice the art of not taking yourself so seriously.

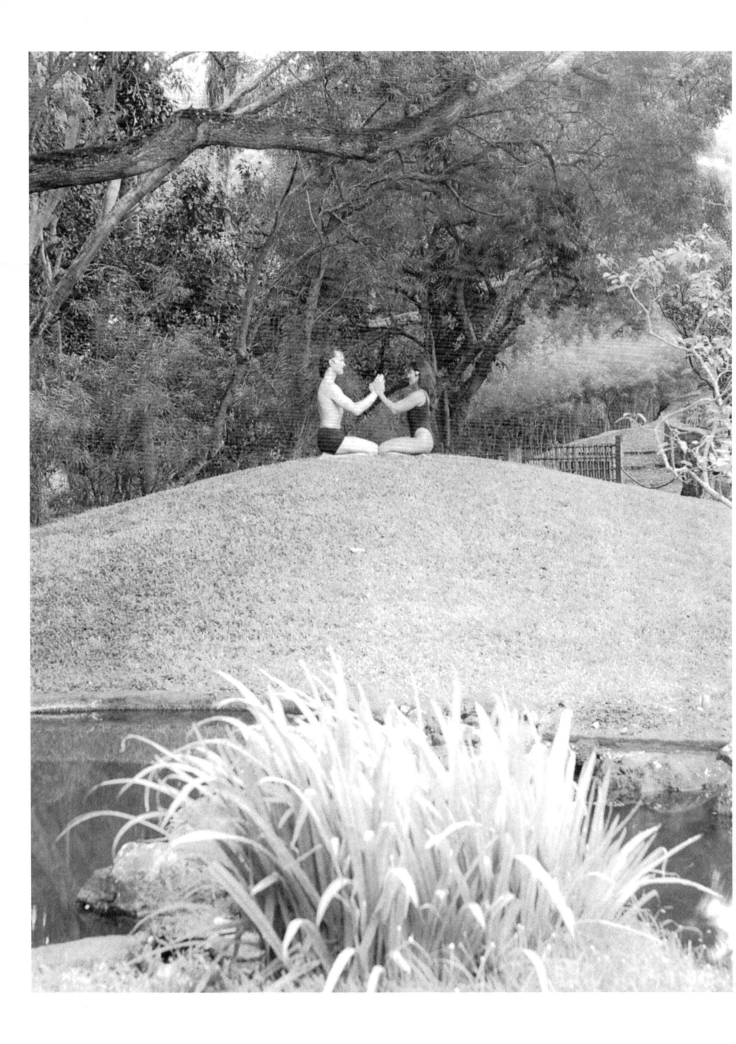

Epilogue

The Quiet Space

"A lamp does not flicker in a place where no winds blow; so it is with a yogi, who controls his mind, intellect, and self, being absorbed in the spirit within him. When the restlessness of the mind, intellect, and self is stilled through the practice of yoga, the yogi by the grace of the Spirit within himself finds fulfillment. Then he knows the joy eternal."

—Krishna speaking to Arjuna in *Bhagavad Gita*

As we have said before, the practice of Partner Yoga is ultimately a journey back to your true self. Through Partner Yoga, you have explored, moved your body, stretched your mind, and opened your heart. And now, we want to invite you to take your experience a little bit deeper. We want to invite you to move toward a place that is beyond movement, beyond thought, to the most sacred place in Partner Yoga—the quiet space.

We live in a time of perpetual clamor. If you were to listen closely inside a typical home, you would hear the low hum of a refrigerator, microwave, and computer, and the buzz of florescent lights. You would hear phones ringing, answering machines beeping, and pots and pans clanking. You would notice clocks ticking and faucets leaking, and hear the subtle drone of a nearby highway. These are a few of the ambient sounds that create the sound track for a 21st-century day: a compilation we have come to call white noise. Our culture has become so accustomed to this noise that the thought of complete silence is almost haunting. In fact, silence is seen as a void that is better off filled with something of substance: conversation, television, radio, anything. For a chunk of money, you can even buy silence from a local radio station and fill it with whatever you choose.

There is something about silence, though—a presence that seems to remain pure, despite our most zealous efforts to fill it. To discover this presence, observe a day of silence. Choose a 24-hour period when you can go through your day without speaking, and make a commitment to yourself to not talk under any circumstances. This simple exercise will do wonders for increasing your sensitivity and inner awareness. "All profound things and emotions of things are preceded and attended by Silence," Herman Melville once said. Silence is present behind everything we do (and all the noise we make in the process). Silence is the underlying force that unites us. Silence exposes our weaknesses and shows us who we really are. Silence is intimate. Perhaps that is why we are only willing to share silence with select people. In silence there is no hiding behind the veil of words or the distraction of sounds. There is only Truth.

As you may have noted, we have dedicated this book to "the Truth finders." For us, the practice of Partner Yoga is, above all else, a process of continually discovering our own unique truth. Each aspect of Partner Yoga plays a unique role in moving us in that direction. The partner postures serve to strengthen our bodies, sharpen our minds, and open our hearts. Practicing breath awareness fortifies the connection between body and mind. And the partner dynamic requires us to be vulnerable, to trust each other, and to surrender to the guidance of our intuition. Ultimately, each of these steps helps us relax and slip gently into the silence and stillness indicative of the quiet space. Traditionally, this is the elusive state that yoga texts (particularly Patanjali's *Yoga Sutra*) refer to as *dhyana*, or absorption into the moment.

One with All Creation

Dhyana is one of the underlying goals of all yoga practice. The word *dhyana* literally means meditation. In the *Yoga Sutra*, meditation is the seventh "limb" in the eight-fold path of yoga, called *ashtanga yoga*. Most people know meditation as a practice done while sitting on a cushion in a cross-legged position, perhaps while counting beads, chanting a sacred mantra, or facing East. Certainly these are forms of meditation. However, meditation is not defined by how you sit or which direction you face. Meditation is a state of being that is not confined to any one form. In fact, every moment is an opportunity to meditate. Partner Yoga becomes meditation when you and your partner are so entirely present in a given posture that everything else fades away. The pose then transforms from something you are doing to something you are becoming. If the pose is balanced and graceful, you become that balance and that grace. If the pose is strong and free, you become that strength and freedom.

In these moments of absorption it is said that we are "yoked" to the underlying force behind all creation. In this place, there are no questions, no opposites, and no struggle; there is only union. This is the essence of yoga. In this quiet space, we are closest to our true selves—we are closest to God.

Resource Guide

Yoga Schools and Training Centers

The following yoga centers are organized under the style of yoga they offer (including the founder of each particular style). There is substantial crossover between yoga schools, and diverse teaching methods are used within each discipline. Contact these centers to find out what types of programs they offer and how to find a yoga center in your area that meets your needs.

Ananda Yoga—Swami Kriyananda
The Expanding Light
Retreat Center at Ananda
14618 Tyler Foote Road
Nevada City, CA 95959
(800) 346-5350 or www.
expandinglight.org

Ashtanga Yoga—K. Pattabhi Jois
Richard Freeman
The Yoga Workshop
2020 21st Street
Boulder, CO 80302

(303) 449-6102 or www.
yogaworkshop.com

Tim Miller
Astanga Yoga Center
118 West E Street
Encinitas, CA 92024
(760) 632-7093 or www.
ashtangayogacenter.com

Bikram Yoga—Bikram Choudhury
Bikram Yoga College of India
8800 Wilshire Boulevard, 2nd Floor
Beverly Hills, CA 90211
(310) 854-5800

Integral Yoga—Swami Satchidananda
Satchidananda Ashram Yogaville
Route One, Box 1720
Buckingham, VA 23921
(800) 858-YOGA, (804) 969-3121,
or www.yogaville.org

Iyengar Yoga—B.K.S. Iyengar
B.K.S. Iyengar Yoga National
Association—USA
1420 Hawthorn Avenue
Boulder, CO 80304
(800) 889-YOGA

Jivamukti—David Life and Sharon Gannon
Jivamukti Yoga Center
404 Lafayette Street, 3rd Floor
New York, NY 10003-6900
(800) 295-6814 or www.jivamuktiyoga.com

Kali Ray Triyoga—Kali Ray
TriYoga International Headquarters
P.O. Box 946
Malibu, CA 90265
(310) 589-0600 or
    www.kaliraytriyoga.com

Kripalu Yoga
Kripalu Center for Yoga and Health
P.O. Box 793
Lenox, MA 01240
(800) 741-7353 or www.kripalu.org

Kundalini Yoga—Yogi Bhajan
International Kundalini Yoga Teachers
    Association
(505) 753-0423 or www.kundaliniyoga.com

Phoenix Rising Yoga Therapy
Phoenix Rising
P.O. Box 819
Housatonic, MA 01236
(800) 288-9642, (413) 232-9800, or
    www.pryt.com

Power Yoga (Based on the principles of Ashtanga Yoga)
Beryl Bender Birch and Thom Birch
The Hard and The Soft Ashtanga Yoga
    Institute
P.O. Box 5009
East Hampton, NY 11937
(212) 661-2895 or www.power-yoga.com

Sivananda Yoga—Swami Vishnu-devananda
Sivananda Ashram Yoga Farm
14651 Ballantree Lane
Grass Valley, CA 95949
(800) 469-9642 or www.sivananda.org

Viniyoga—TKV Desikachar
Gary Kraftsow
The American Viniyoga Institute
P.O.Box 88
Makawao, HI 96768
(808) 572-1414 or www.viniyoga.com

Richard Miller, Ph.D.
Anahata Press
P.O. Box 1673
Sebastopol, CA 95473
(415) 456-3909 or www.nondual.com

White Lotus—
Ganga White and Tracey Rich
White Lotus Foundation
2500 San Marcos Pass
Santa Barbara, CA 93105
(800) 544-FLOW or www.whitelotus.org

Yoga Magazines

Yoga Journal: (800) 600-YOGA or
    www.yogajournal.com; from outside
    the United States, call (760) 796-6549

Yoga International: (800) 253-6243

Yoga Supplies

Inner Dimensions Catalog:
    www.innerdimensions.com

Fish Crane: (800) 959-6116

Bheka Yoga Supplies: (800) 366-4541 or
    www.bheka.com

Living Arts: (800) 254-8464 or
    www.gaiam.com

Glossary

Adho Muka Svanasana: Downward Facing Dog Pose

Ardha Chandrasana: Half Moon Pose

Ardha Matsyendrasana: Half Spinal Twist Pose

Asana: Posture or position. The third limb of the eight-fold path of yoga which involves the practice of techniques to purify the body and focus the mind

Ashtanga yoga: The eight-fold path of yoga as described by the Indian sage, Patanjali

Balasana: Child Pose

Bhujangasana: Cobra Pose

Chakrasana: Wheel Pose

Chandrasana: Moon Pose

Conscious Breathing: The practice of observing the ebb and flow of the breath as a means of calming and focusing the mind

Danurasana: Bow Pose

Dharana: Concentration of the mind; single-pointed focus; the sixth limb in the eight-fold path of yoga

Dhyana: Meditation, or absorption in the moment; a fundamental technique of all yogic practices (the seventh limb in the eight-fold path of yoga)

Diaphragm: The flat sheet of muscle that separates the chest cavity from the abdominal cavity; its movement plays a major role in proper breathing

Dynamic: A state of constant change of movement

Gheranda Samhita: Literally, "Gheranda's Compendium"; a late 17th-century manual on hatha yoga

Halasana: Plow Pose

Hatha Yoga: From "ha," meaning sun, "tha," meaning moon, and yoga, meaning union; the practice of hatha yoga uses physical and mental exercises to balance the opposing forces within the body

230

Hatha Yoga Pradipika: Literally, "Light on the Forceful Yoga"; one of the most widely used classical texts on yoga; written in the mid-14th century, the text seeks to integrate the physical disciplines with the higher spiritual goals of yoga

Hinduism: The religious and social system of the Hindus from the land of Indus, or India

Janu Sirsasana: Head to Knee Pose

Jnana mudra: The seal of wisdom; formed by touching the tips of the thumb and forefinger together

Karma Yoga: The yoga of self-transcending action; a path of yoga, introduced more than 2,000 years ago in the famous *Bhagavad Gita*, which encourages an active life of service

Kundalini: "Serpent power"; the divine cosmic energy (shakti) that lies dormant in each individual. Many schools of yoga conceptualize the kundalini as a feminine serpent coiled 3½ times at the base of the spine. The rising of the kundalini up the astral spine (shushumna nadi) toward the head is said to open the door to liberation

Matsyasana: Fish Pose

Meditation: The elevated state of consciousness characterized by stillness and inner peace

Namaste: A salutation among yogis meaning, "I honor the deepest and highest Truth residing within you. When you are in that place within yourself, and I am in that place within myself, we are one"

Natarajasana: Pose of Siva, the Cosmic Dancer

Naturopathic Medicine: The science, philosophy, and art of using natural substances and modalities to address the cause of disease and restore harmony and well-being

Navasana: Boat Pose

Padahastasana: Hand to Foot Pose

Padmasana: Lotus Pose

Parivritta Trikonasana: Revolved Triangle Pose

Paschimottanasana: Seated Forward Bend Pose

Patanjali: An Indian sage famous for his contributions (namely the *Yoga Sutra*) to the field of yoga. He is believed to have lived around the second century CE

Prana: Vital life force or breath. The subtle energy referred to as *ki* in Japanese tradition, *qi* or *chi* in Chinese medicine, and *mana* in Hawaiian

Pranayama: "Prana" is life force and "yama" is control. Pranayama denotes any yogic technique used to control life force. Yogic breathing exercises are typically called pranayams, and the practice of pranayama is integral to both yoga and meditation

Sarvangasana: Shoulderstand Pose

Upavista Konasana: Seated Angel Pose

Utkatasana: Camel Pose

Uttanasana: Standing Forward Bend Pose

Utthita Hasta Padangustasana: Extended Hand to Foot Pose

Utthita Parsvakonasana: Extended Lateral Angle Pose

Utthita Trikonasana: Extended Triangle Pose

Virabhadrasana: Warrior Pose

Vriksasana: Tree Pose

Yoga Korunta: An ancient yoga manual allegedly inscribed on palm leaves

Yoga Sutra: Aphorisms on yoga; one of the classical texts on yoga, consisting of four chapters with a total of 195 aphorisms, written around the 2nd century CE by the famous sage Patanjali

Bibliography

Bach, Richard. *Jonathan Livingston Seagull*. New York: Avon Books, 1970.

Birch, Beryl Bender. *Power Yoga*. New York: Fireside, 1995.

Cousins, Norman. *Anatomy of an Illness*. New York: W.W. Norton and Company, 1979.

Cushman, Anne. "New Light on Yoga." *Yoga Journal* (July/August 1999): 44–49.

Dawson, Larry. *Touch, Not Necessarily Sex*. Hawaii: Bodissage, 1987.

Desai, Amrit. *Kripalu Yoga: Meditation in Motion*. Boston: Kripalu Publications, 1985.

Desikachar, T.K.V. *The Heart of Yoga: Developing a Personal Practice (Revised Edition)*. Rochester, Vt.: Inner Traditions International, 1999.

Feuerstein, Georg. *The Shambhala Encyclopedia of Yoga*. Boston: Shambhala Publications, 1997.

Feuerstein, Georg, and Stephan Bodian. *Living Yoga*. New York: Tarcher/Putnam, 1993.

Fisher, Robert. *The Knight in Rusty Armor*. Hollywood: Melvin Powers Wilshire Book Company, 1990.

Franklin, Eric. *Dynamic Alignment through Imagery*. Champaign, Ill.: Human Kinetics, 1996.

Hanh, Thich Nhat. *The Miracle of Mindfulness*. Boston: Beacon Press, 1987.

Hanna, Thomas. *Somatics*. Reading, Mass.: Perseus, 1988.

Iyengar, B.K.S. *Light on Pranayama: The Yogic Art of Breathing*. New York: Crossroad, 1997.

Iyengar, B.K.S. *Light on Yoga (Revised Edition)*. New York: Schocken, 1979.

Koren, Leonard. *Wabi-Sabi for Artists, Designers, Poets, and Philosophers*. Berkeley: Stone Bridge Press, 1994.

Kriyananda, Swami (J. Donald Walters). *14 Steps to Higher Awareness*. Nevada City, Calif.: Ananda Church of Self-Realization, 1989.

Montagu, Ashley. *Touching: The Human Significance of the Skin (3rd Edition)*. New York: Harper and Row, 1986.

Reid, Darlene W., and Gail Dechman. "Considerations When Testing and Training the Respiratory Muscles." *Physical Therapy* 75(11), Nov. 1995.

Sivananda Yoga Vedanta Center. *Yoga Mind and Body*. New York: DK Publishing, 1996.

White, Ganga. *Double Yoga*. New York: Penguin, 1981.

Index

Boldface page references indicate illustrations and photographs. Underscored page references indicate boxed text.

E

F

G

About the Authors and Photographer

Cain Carroll is a certified yoga instructor with a diverse background in wrestling, martial arts, dance, and meditation. His unique approach to yoga reflects a multicultural, multidisciplinary influence, which he uses to create an inspiring arena for personal enrichment, cultural understanding, and global transformation. He lives and teaches in Hawaii.

Lori Kimata, N.D., comes from a rich background in dance, music, and art, which she integrates into her profession as a naturopathic physician, midwife, yoga instructor, and international guest lecturer. She has recently returned to her native *Hawai'i* to cultivate an open, sacred space to practice the "Art of Living Your Love."

Ken Gray has been a professional photographer for 30 years. Gray began photographing yoga postures in 1988, marrying his passion for both yoga and photography. Gray's other photographic interests include helicopter aerial photography, tribal and native elders and cultures, children, and landscapes.

For more information on Partner Yoga, visit the authors' Web site at www.partneryoga.com.

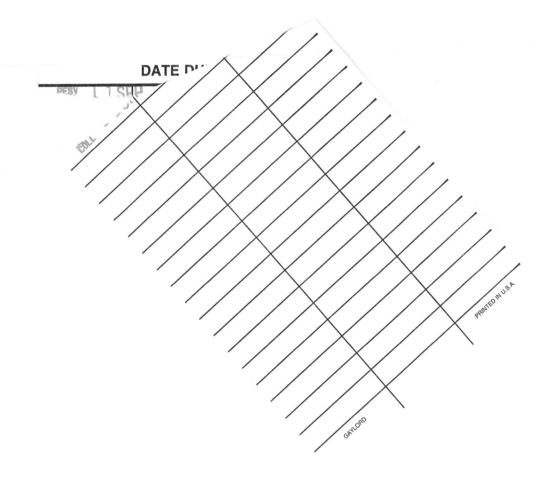

DATE DUE

PRINTED IN U.S.A.

GAYLORD

Breinigsville, PA USA
19 January 2011
253621BV00001B/159-162/P

9 781605 296999